Preface

This, the first volume in a new series of illustrated, specialised diagnostic problems, is intended for all candidates revising for undergraduate or post-graduate examinations in paediatrics. In common with all clinical specialities, correct diagnosis in paediatrics is largely dependent upon careful history and examination but the possibilities for 'spot' diagnosis do exist. The problems posed in this book vary in difficulty and the answers vary in depth and scope. We estimate that an under-graduate should be able to solve a third of the set questions, while the average candidate for the DCH examination is expected to answer a further third. As the slides and questions are similar to those prepared for the MRCP (Paediatric) examination, it is hoped that the book as a whole will be particularly useful to such students and, also, will prove to be a stimulus to further reading for both undergraduates and postgraduates. The authors would like to thank our local MRCP candidates who served, unknowingly in many respects, as the moderators of some of the questions.

Acknowledgements

We wish to thank the Departments of Medical Illustration at the Northern General Hospital and Royal Hallamshire Hospital, Sheffield, for their assistance with photography and duplication. We are grateful to Mrs G Wilson for her patient typing of the text and we thank Dr R A Primhak for helpful discussion. The generous co-operation of the following colleagues who provided slides is appreciated:

Dr A W Boon
Mr J A S Dickson
Professor B I Duerden
Dr M B Duggan
Dr J M King
Dr R K Levick
Dr J S Lilleyman
Mr A E MacKinnon
Dr J E Oliver
Dr R G Pearse
Dr M Placzek

Dr D A Price
Dr B L Priestley
Dr R A Primhak
Dr M F Smith
Mr R Spicer
Professor L Spitz
Dr G M Steiner
Dr L S Taitz
Dr S Variend
Dr J K H Wales
Dr G Whincup

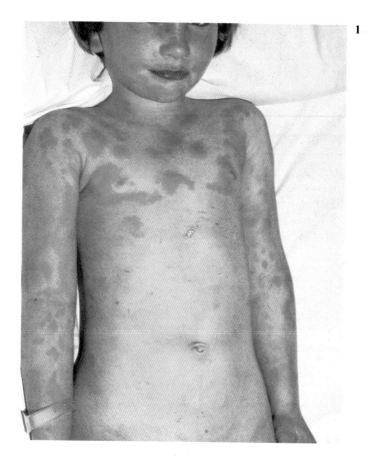

A boy was admitted to hospital the previous day with
fever, malaise and this obvious skin rash.
(a) What is the name of the rash?
(b) What part of the body is characteristically avoided
in this eruption?
(c) What is the treatment of choice?

2

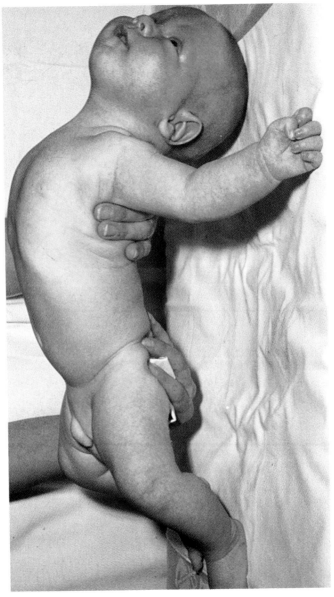

2 This infant felt floppy when handled by the nurse. Name five possible causes of such floppiness.

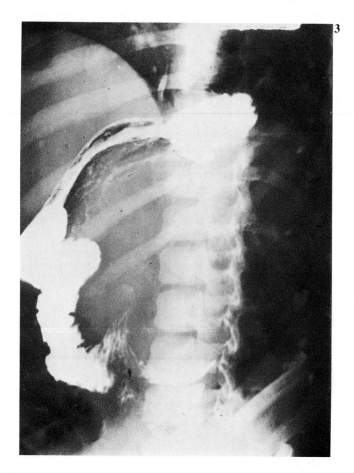

3 Radiograph shows contrast medium in the stomach during the course of a barium meal examination.
(a) What abnormality is shown?
(b) What is the commonest cause of this abnormality?
(c) What is the most likely clinical presentation?

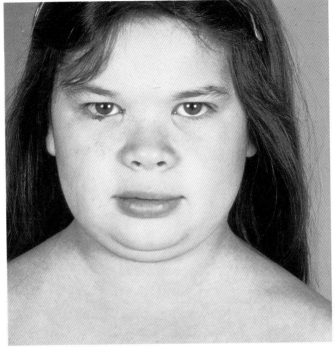

4 A seven-year-old girl was referred from the School Health Service because of short stature. Her progress in school was satisfactory and her parents had no specific worries. Her weight was on the 50th centile, her height was on the 3rd. Both parents were on the 75th centile for height.
(a) What is the diagnosis?
(b) In children presenting in this way, is school progress normally satisfactory?
(c) State two investigations which will help you to arrive at a diagnosis.

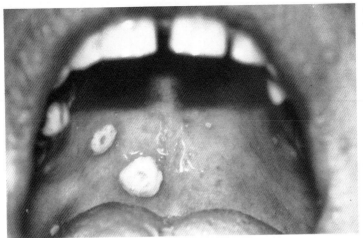

5 A nine-year-old boy was admitted to hospital, having been feverish and systemically unwell for two days. Physical examination was within normal limits except for the lesions shown here and four macules on the neck.
(a) What is the likely diagnosis?
(b) State three ways in which the diagnosis may be confirmed.

6 Radiograph from an intravenous pyelogram.
(a) What condition is apparent?
(b) What is the likely cause of the gastric dilation?

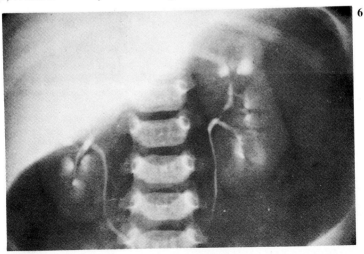

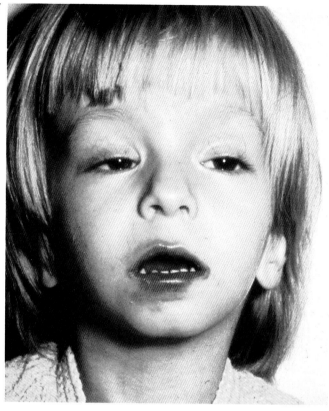

7 A child has a diagnostically characteristic facies.
(a) What condition does he have?
(b) Name three other characteristics of the condition.

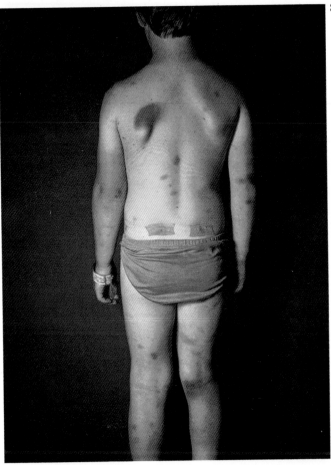

8 A stocky seven-year-old boy was referred to the hospital as an emergency by the Social Services Department. The family had been followed for several years because of poor home circumstances. His teacher and neighbours had complained that the boy had excessive bruising. On examination the bruises shown were the only abnormal findings. Investigations showed the platelet count to be normal, the prothrombin time and thrombin time were normal, but the bleeding time was 17 minutes. No history of drug ingestion could be elicited.
(a) What is the most likely diagnosis?
(b) Name two confirmatory tests.

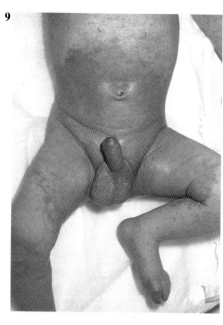

9 A mother presented at an infant welfare clinic with her three-month-old infant, complaining that he had a nappy rash.

(a) What is the cause of the nappy rash?

(b) Name two organisms which commonly cause superinfection.

(c) What other part of the body characteristically may be affected?

10 A three-year-old was brought to the Accident and Emergency Department because she refused to swallow and was drooling.

(a) What condition is demonstrated?

(b) What is responsible for the acute inflammation and ulceration of the throat?

(c) What treatment is available?

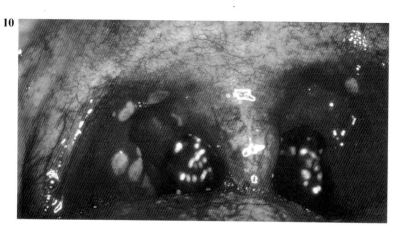

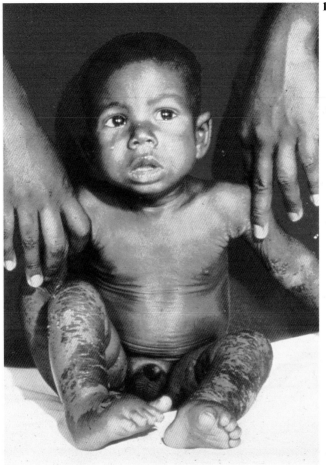

11 A 15-month-old boy was brought to the Government Hospital in a developing country by his elder sister. He weighed 6.3kg but no other symptoms were proffered. Physical examination showed him to have oedema of the legs, hyper- and hypopigmented skin and thin friable reddish hair.

(a) What condition is he suffering from?
(b) Which age group is most commonly affected?
(c) Name two causes for hepatomegaly in this child.

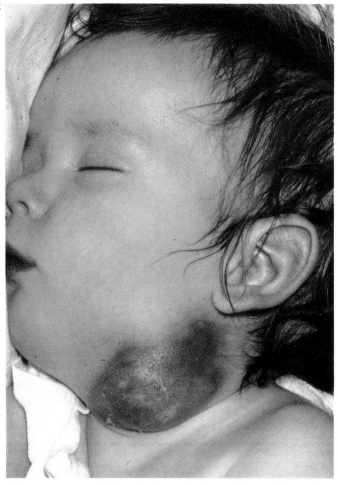

12 An 18-month-old infant with bilateral swelling of the neck was taken to his general practitioner, who diagnosed tonsillitis. Five days later he was brought to hospital with the swelling as shown. Examination of the mouth revealed pus at the opening of Stensen's duct.
(a) What condition is illustrated?
(b) In which common illness may this be a complication?
(c) What is the most common causative organism?

13 This is a child with the characteristic facies of a mucopolysaccharidosis. In the evaluation of such a patient, state three important features in the history and clinical examination which may help in differentiating between the Hunter and the Hurler syndrome.

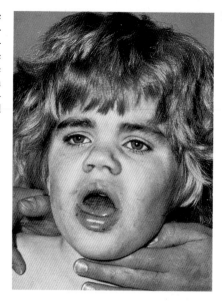

14 A baby was taken to the family doctor with a rash around the mouth. The lesions were swabbed but no organism could be cultured.
(a) What is the likely diagnosis?
(b) What is the explanation for the colour of the lesions?
(c) What treatment may be of benefit?

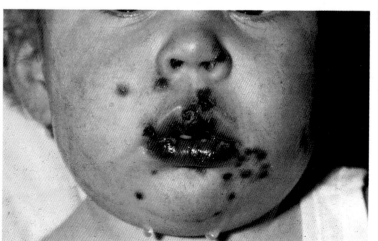

15

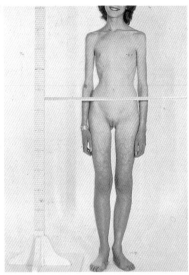

15 A 17-year-old girl had no symptoms but her parents were concerned about her.
(a) Name two abnormalities illustrated.
(b) State two possible explanations for the clinical abnormalities.

16 An eight-year-old girl presented with a five-month history of weight loss, abdominal pain and intermittent diarrhoea. Blood had been noticed in her stools on two occasions. She also complained of a sore mouth.
(a) What is the likely diagnosis?
(b) What abnormality is shown?
(c) What is the investigation of choice to help to prove the diagnosis?

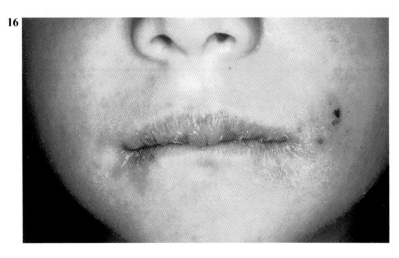

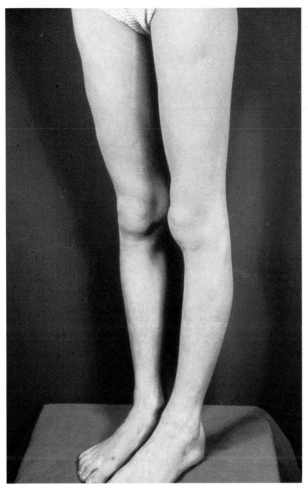

17 A diabetic girl complained of the shape of her thighs.
(a) What abnormality is illustrated?
(b) State two ways in which the condition may be treated.

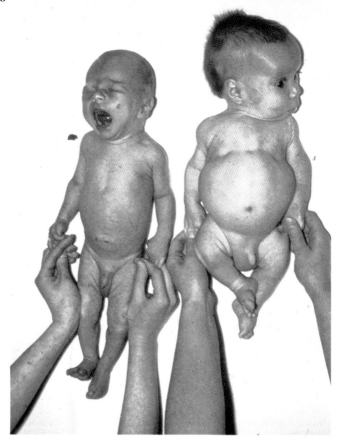

18 The infant on the left of these two newborn infants of the same gestational age is normal.
(a) What condition does the other infant have?
(b) What is the mode of inheritance?
(c) What spinal lesion is often a feature of this condition?

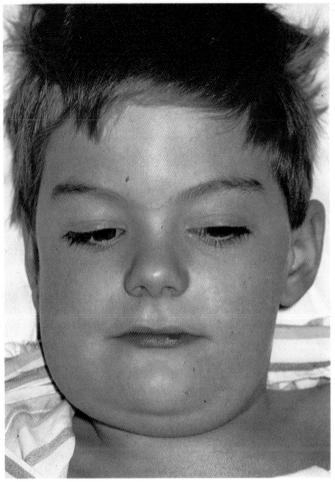

19 A nine-year-old boy developed bilateral parotid swelling and neck stiffness following a two-day history of pain in the angle of the jaw and general malaise. Examination of the CSF showed 400 lymphocytes per mm^3.
(a) What condition is the boy suffering from?
(b) What may be revealed by clinical examination of the throat?
(c) Name two further complications of the primary illness.

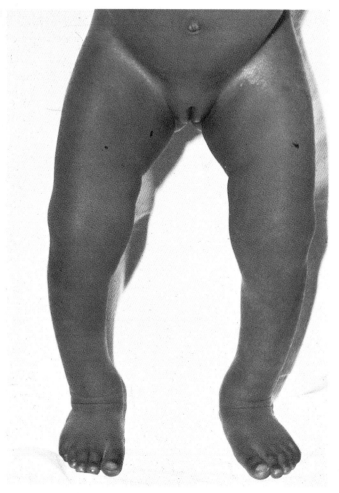

20 A health visitor noticed the features shown in a routine examination of toddlers attending a nursery.
(a) What gave cause for concern?
What is the likely explanation for the finding:
(b) in an asymptomatic child?
(c) in a child reared in a poor social environment?
(d) in a child known to be suffering from chronic renal disease?

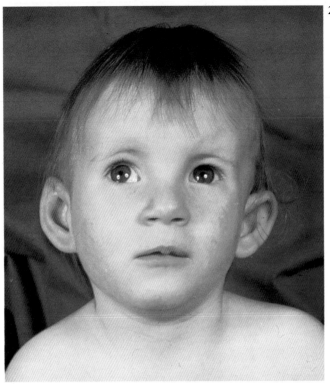

21 A three-year-old boy was referred because of psychomotor delay. Chromosomal examination revealed a deletion of the short arm of chromosome 5.
(a) What is the diagnosis?
(b) Name two characteristic features shown which suggest the diagnosis.
(c) What is the prognosis for height and longevity?

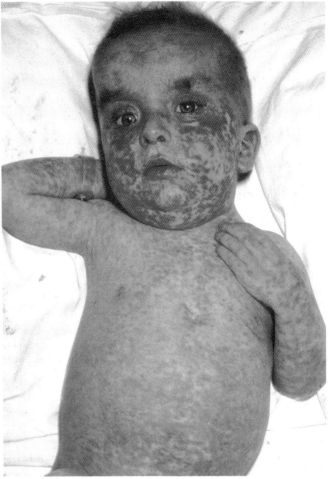

22 A six-month-old infant was admitted unwell, with a fever and rash.
(a) Which exanthem is he suffering from?
(b) State three complications of the illness.
(c) If the child developed the rash in an open hospital ward, how should the other patients be managed?

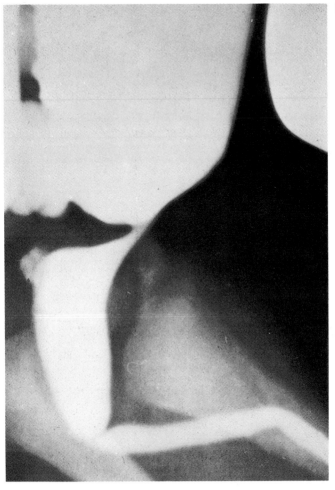

23 Radiograph shows a micturating cystourethrogram.
(a) What condition is illustrated?
(b) How may this present clinically?
(c) To prove the diagnosis, how should the micturating cystourethrogram be performed?

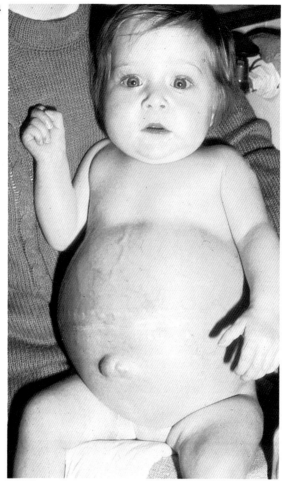

24 (a) Name three clinical abnormalities visible in this nine-month-old child.
(b) What is the likely cause of these abnormalities?
(c) What is the treatment of choice?

25 This newborn baby shows a striking abnormality.
(a) What is it?
(b) Name three conditions with which this abnormality may be associated.

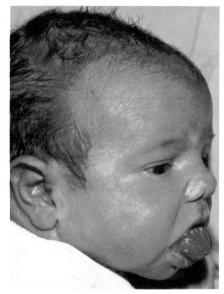

26 This two-year-old presented to the Accident and Emergency Department after a choking attack followed by a six-hour history of acute dyspnoea.
(a) Name three abnormalities seen on the chest radiograph.
(b) What may be the cause?

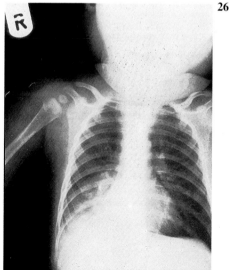

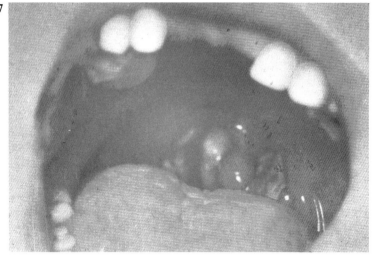

27 (a) What abnormality is apparent?
(b) Name three organisms which may be responsible for this clinical finding.

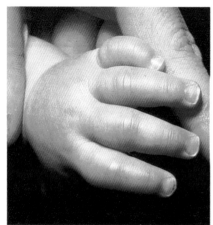

28 This infant had a painful hand.
(a) What abnormality is shown?
(b) Name two causes for the clinical abnormality.

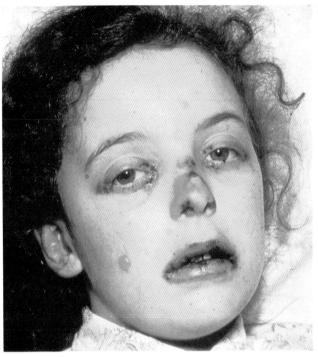

29 This eight-year-old girl had been treated with cotrimoxazole for her first attack of urinary tract infection. Four days later she presented at the hospital toxic, feverish and with the lesions shown.
(a) What condition is she suffering from?
(b) With what infection may this condition be associated in other patients?

30

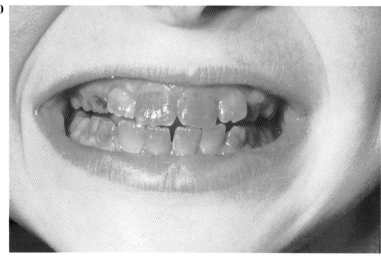

30 (a) What abnormality is shown?
(b) Name two causes of this condition.
(c) After what age is this unlikely to occur?

31

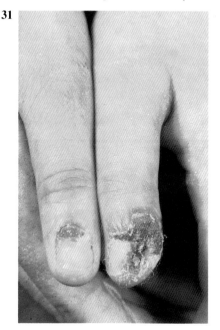

31 A 12-year-old girl was receiving immunosuppressive therapy for a renal disorder. The lesion on her finger had been steadily worsening over the previous two weeks. Initially, her parents felt that it was due to her chewing her nails but later they sought medical advice.
(a) What is the diagnosis?
(b) What is the treatment of choice?

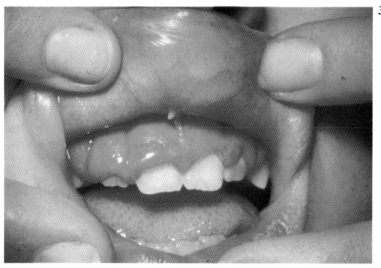

32 (a) What abnormality is seen in the mouth of this child?
(b) Name two causes for this abnormality.

33 An eight-year-old girl presented to her family doctor with a history of fever, sore throat and general malaise, for which she was treated with an antibiotic. Several days later she developed the rash shown.
(a) What is the rash due to?
(b) What was the likely presenting complaint?
(c) Which two laboratory investigations might help in confirming the diagnosis?

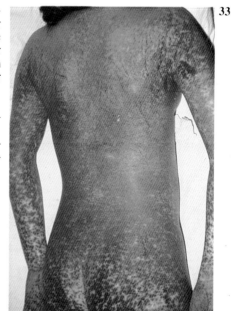

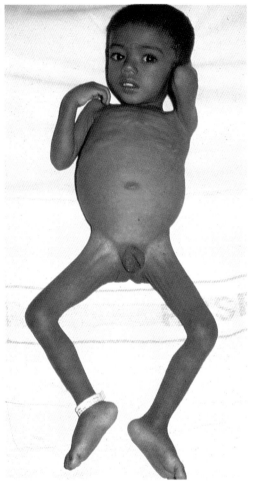

34 This two-year-old boy was seen in a developing country. His height and weight were both well below the 3rd centile. He was said to have thrived until the birth of his sibling one year earlier.
(a) What is the diagnosis?
(b) What features may this condition have in common with hypothyroidism?
(c) Why has the birth of his sibling precipitated this condition?

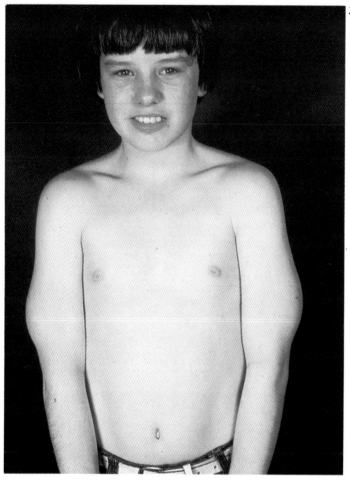

35 (a) What caused the lumps on this boy's arms?
(b) How may they affect the overall management of his chronic condition?

36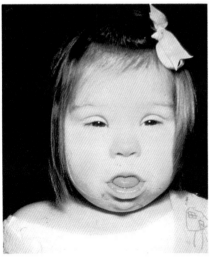

36 A 15-month-old girl presented with a history of lethargy, developmental delay and obesity. She had been passed as normal at birth.
(a) What is the diagnosis?
(b) How may this be confirmed by a single laboratory test?
(c) What is a radiograph of the wrist likely to show?

37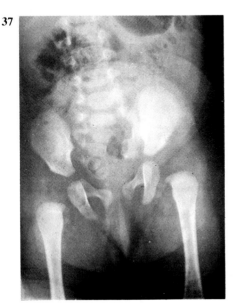

37 A two-day-old infant was referred because of an abdominal mass. On examination he was noted to have a smooth suprapubic mass, dribbling of urine and a patulous anus. A cleft was present over the left side of the sacrum.
(a) What is demonstrated in the radiograph?
(b) What is the abdominal mass?
(c) What is the diagnosis?

38 The facies of this newborn infant are characteristic of a chromosomal anomaly.
(a) What is the condition called and which chromosomes are abnormal?
(b) What abnormality of the feet is often seen?
(c) What is the long term prognosis?

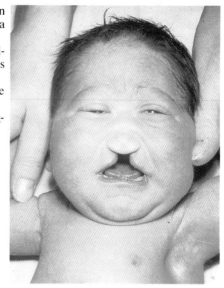

39 A four-year-old girl presented to Outpatients because of the concern of the School Medical Officer. The parents had no worry about her. Careful clinical examination failed to reveal any abnormality other than that shown.
(a) What abnormality is apparent?
(b) What is the likely diagnosis?
(c) Name two investigations which may help in the evaluation of the condition.

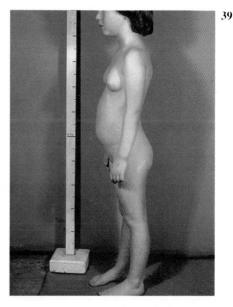

40

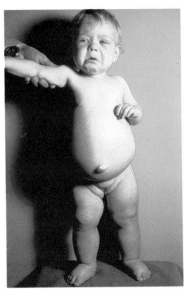

40 A two-year-old child presented with generalised oedema; examination of the urine showed marked proteinuria but no haematuria.

(a) What condition is she likely to suffer from?

(b) What percentage of such children will relapse?

(c) What is the treatment of choice?

41 An eight-year-old boy was submitted to a slit lamp examination as part of the spectrum of investigations of his ataxia. The ocular findings are characteristic of a specific diagnosis.

(a) What is the diagnosis?

(b) What is the treatment of choice for this diagnosis?

(c) How is this condition inherited?

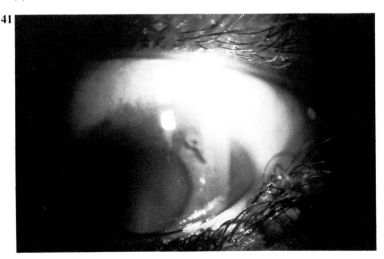

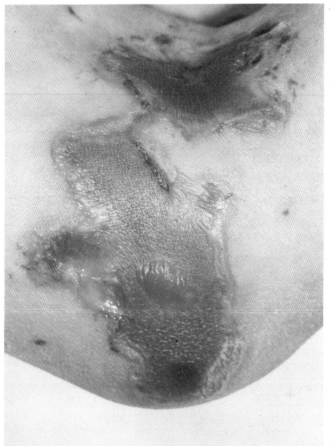

42 A child was admitted to hospital moribund suffering from septicaemia. The skin lesions shown appeared over the next 48 hours during treatment in the intensive care unit.

(a) What is the nature of the lesions?

(b) What is the commonest cause in childhood for this sequence of events?

43

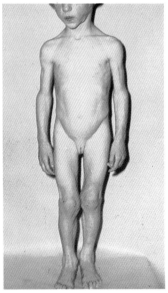

43 A five-year-old girl was asymptomatic, but was brought to hospital for specialist consultation because of her body habitus.
(a) What abnormality is shown?
(b) What is the likely diagnosis?

44 A barium meal was performed on an 18-month-old boy who presented with a history of persistent vomiting.
(a) What abnormality is demonstrated on this radiograph?
(b) Name three other common presentations for this condition in childhood.

45 A five-year-old girl presented with recurrent abdominal pain and bloody diarrhoea.
(a) What abnormalities are apparent in the perineal region?
(b) The lesions and the history are characteristic of which condition?
(c) What is the investigation of choice?

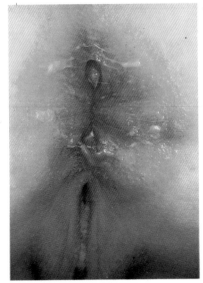

46 Skull radiograph of a child who had a history of focal convulsions.
(a) What abnormality is shown?
(b) What is the mode of inheritance of the underlying condition?

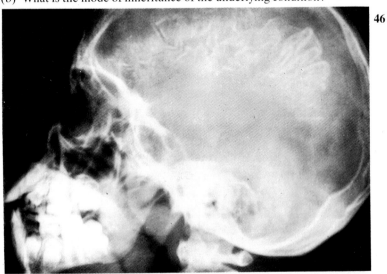

47

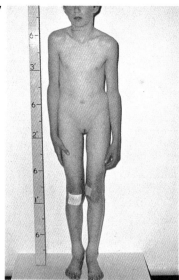

47 (a) What are the striking abnormalities apparent in this six-year-old symptomless girl?
(b) What is the differential diagnosis?
(c) How does the inheritance of the two principal conditions differ?

48 A newborn infant shows a characteristic abnormality.
(a) What is it?
(b) Name two syndromes in which this abnormality may be found.

48

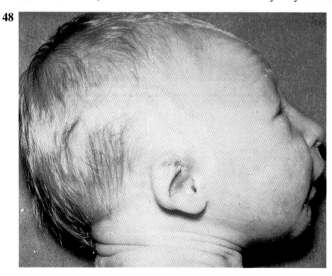

49 A six-year-old boy was referred by his school doctor because of pubic hair.
(a) Name two other abnormalities demonstrated.
(b) Name two conditions that could cause this.

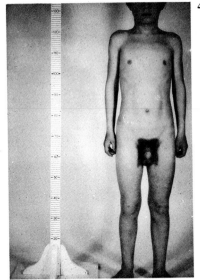

50 A ten-year-old boy of gipsy parents presented to hospital with a three-day history of fever, malaise and sore throat. On the day of admission his voice suddenly became high-pitched and he started to regurgitate fluid through his nose. On examination his temperature was 37.5°C, heart rate 160/min. and he had an exudative tonsillitis, cervical lymphadenitis and marked oedema of the neck.
(a) What is the diagnosis?
(b) What treatment is indicated?
(c) Name two laboratory tests of value.

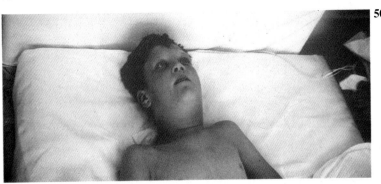

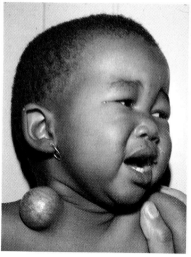

51 A child of African parents presented with a three months' history of progressive malaise, weight loss and nocturnal cough. The swelling was first noticed one month after the onset of symptoms. Examination revealed an unwell child with an enlarged inflamed right tonsil but no other abnormality.

(a) What is the most likely diagnosis?

(b) Name two investigations that may be useful.

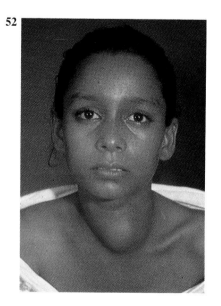

52 A 13-year-old girl presented with a swelling in the neck.

(a) What is this likely to be?

(b) What manoeuvres on clinical examination confirm the anatomical diagnosis?

(c) What is the treatment of choice?

53 A child was noted to have a neck swelling at school entry examination which moved when she stuck out her tongue. Between referral and attendance at Outpatients she developed malaise, a swinging fever and tenderness over the lump.
(a) What is the diagnosis?
(b) What is the treatment of choice?

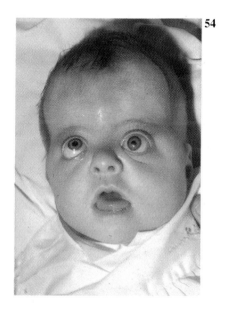

54 (a) What is the diagnosis in this infant?
(b) What is the cause of the abnormal clinical findings?

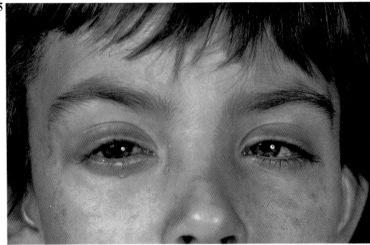

55 A five-year-old girl was under neurological supervision for progressive ataxia. At a clinic visit her mother pointed out the facial rash which had not responded to topical ointment prescribed by her general practitioner.
(a) What is the diagnosis?
(b) What is the mode of inheritance?
(c) Name two serious long term complications.

56 An eight-month-old child from a socially deprived background presented with the above lesion and similar lesions on the abdomen, buttocks and soles of the feet.
(a) What is the most likely diagnosis?
(b) What two investigations must be carried out in these circumstances?

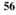 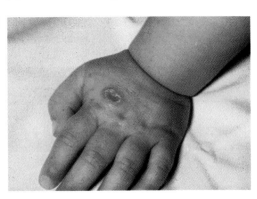

57 (a) What syndrome is demonstrated?
(b) Name two clinical problems associated with this.

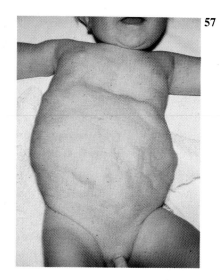

58 A little girl presented with acute urinary retention.
(a) What abnormality is shown?
(b) What age range is most commonly affected?
(c) How is this condition treated?

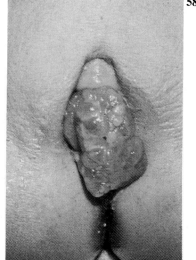

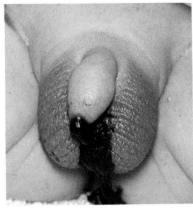

59 Concern was expressed about this 22-hour-old baby boy.
(a) What abnormality is shown?
(b) What is this due to?
(c) What is the prognosis for long term continence of stool?

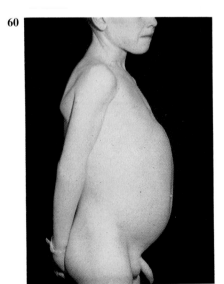

60 A ten-year-old boy presented with a history of gross constipation since early life. Treatment with laxatives had been largely ineffective.
(a) What abnormality is shown?
(b) What is the most likely diagnosis?
(c) What is the treatment of choice?

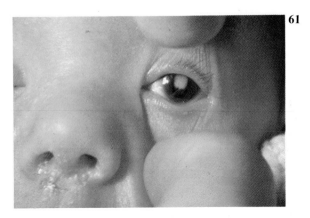

61 (a) What abnormality is apparent in this one-month-old infant?
(b) Name three possible causes in this particular case.

62 This is the anterior abdominal wall of a 12-year-old girl one week after appendicectomy which was carried out following a history of intermittent abdominal pain and vomiting for two months.
(a) What is the likely primary pathology?
(b) Name important aspects of immediate and long term management.

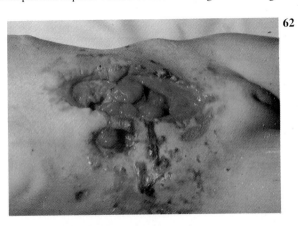

63

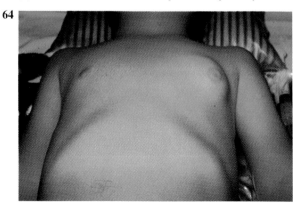

63 (a) What abnormality is shown?
(b) What is the commonest reason for this?

64 This is a 13-year-old boy.
(a) What abnormality is demonstrated?
(b) What is the treatment of choice?
(c) Name two other causes, apart from puberty.

64

65 (a) What abnormality is shown?
(b) What is the commonest cause of this?
(c) What other bone may be abnormal?

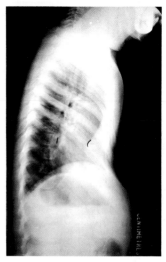

65

66 (a) What abnormality is shown in this nine-month-old infant?
(b) In what syndrome may this occur?
(c) What is the treatment of choice?

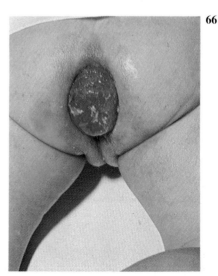

66

67

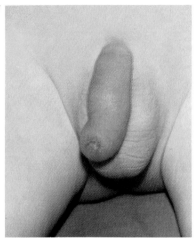

67 This boy presented with acute difficulty in micturition.
(a) What condition is shown?
(b) What is the treatment of choice?

68

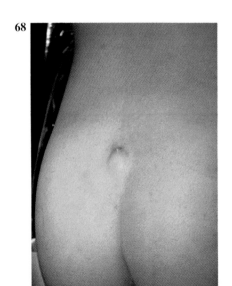

68 An eight-year-old child presented with acute paralysis of both legs associated with loss of bladder and bowel control. The lesion shown had been present since birth, but had been asymptomatic.
(a) What is the lesion?
(b) What emergency investigation should be carried out?

69 (a) What abnormalities are seen in this newborn infant?
(b) What is the diagnosis?
(c) What is the prognosis for long term normal development?

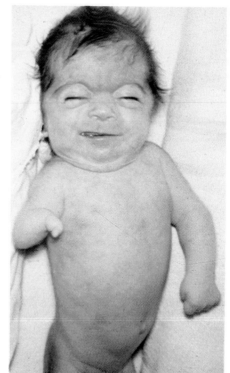

70 (a) What abnormality is apparent?
(b) Which age group is most commonly affected?
(c) If this abnormality occurs unilaterally, what is the commonest cause?

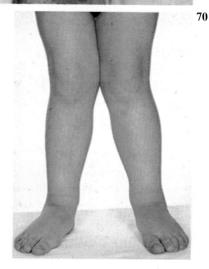

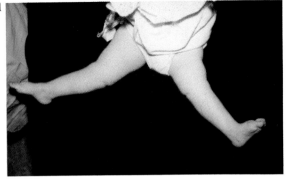

71 (a) What skeletal abnormality does this infant manifest?
(b) Name three possible causes of the abnormality.

72 (a) What condition is this?
(b) What is the cause?
(c) What clinical symptoms and signs may be associated with this abnormality?

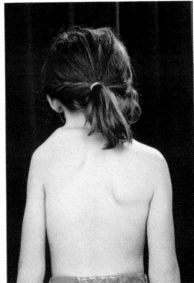

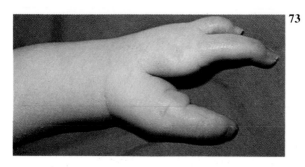

73 (a) What defect is this?
(b) In what syndrome is this abnormality characteristic?
(c) With which other feature is it associated?

74 A three-year-old boy presented to a rural clinic in Africa.
(a) What is the most likely cause of his swelling?
(b) With which virus is this swelling associated?
(c) What other tumour may mimic this swelling?

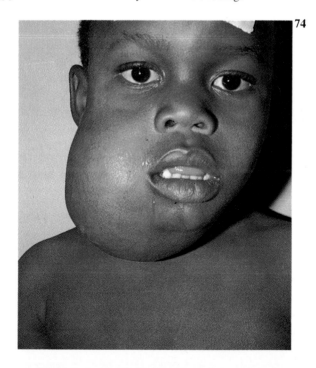

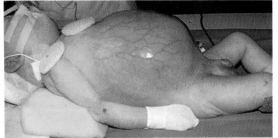

75 (a) Describe the abnormality apparent in this five-day-old infant.
(b) Name four causes.

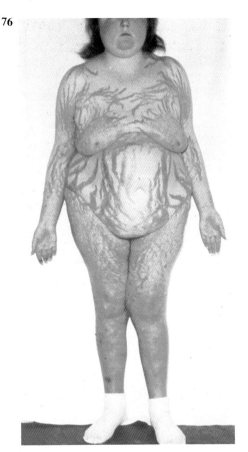

76 A 10-year-old girl presented with distressing obesity, and a careful history failed to reveal any evidence of drug ingestion.
(a) What is the likely diagnosis?
(b) What effect is this likely to have on her adult height?
(c) What is the commonest aetiology in this child?

77 A midwife found it impossible to take a rectal temperature reading after removing a meconium-filled nappy.
(a) What is the likely explanation for this?
(b) What is the treatment of choice?

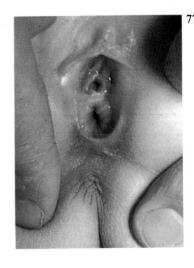

78 (a) What abnormality is seen in this baby's facial structure?
(b) With what tumour is this phenomenon sometimes associated?

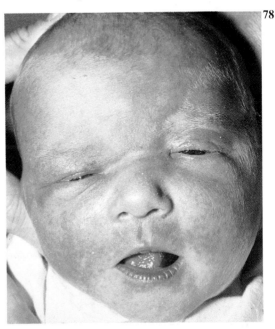

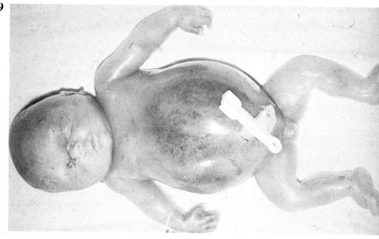

79 (a) What abnormality does this stillborn infant show?
(b) Name two non-haematological causes of this condition.

80 These infants are twins photographed within one hour of birth.
(a) What condition is illustrated?
(b) Which of the twins is at greater risk?
(c) What treatment is required?

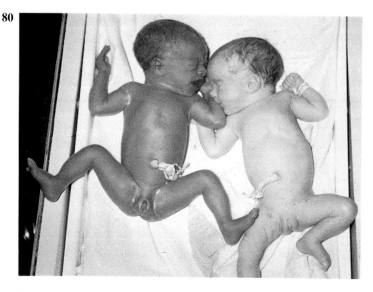

81 An 18-month-old boy was born large-for-dates and macroglossia was apparent at birth. He was operated on in the immediate neonatal period for exomphalos.
(a) What condition is he suffering from?
(b) What abnormality of the ears is characteristic of this syndrome?
(c) In what way may such infants have a life-threatening crisis?

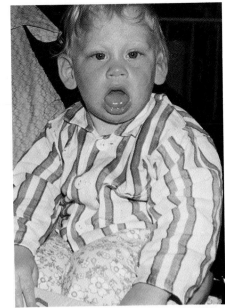

82 A newborn infant was noted to have this lesion present from birth. Name three possible diagnoses.

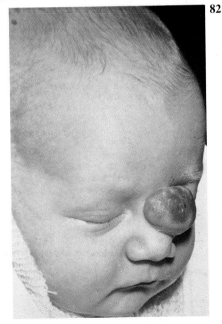

83

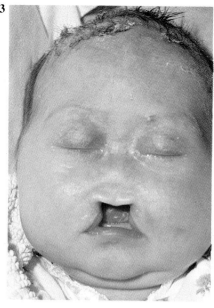

83 (a) What clinical abnormalities are shown in this newborn infant?

(b) Of what condition is the face characteristic?

(c) What abnormality of the brain may coexist?

(d) What may be revealed by examination of the chromosomes?

84

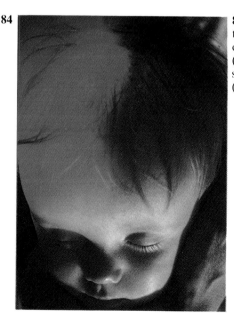

84 These are the results of transillumination of the skull of a three-month-old infant.

(a) What abnormality is shown?

(b) Name two possible causes.

85 (a) What abnormality is shown in this postmortem specimen of a neonatal brain?
(b) Name three factors that predispose to this.
(c) Name two long term complications in survivors.

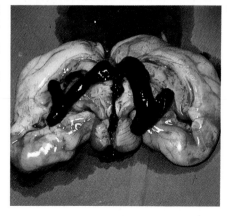

86 A four-week-old infant was the third child of healthy, unrelated parents. Pregnancy and delivery were uncomplicated and the baby was discharged home well at the age of 48 hours. He presented with a lump in the neck.
(a) What is the diagnosis?
(b) What is the treatment of choice?
(c) How commonly does this occur following uncomplicated delivery?

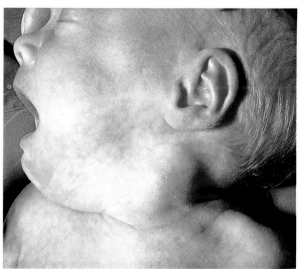

87

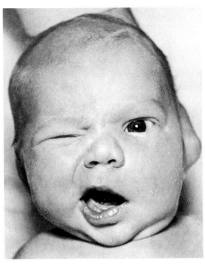

87 (a) What abnormality is shown?
(b) What is the prognosis?

88 An infant, the second child of a 17-year-old unmarried mother, presented at 18 hours of age with the abnormalities shown.
(a) What is wrong?
(b) What is the likely causative organism?
(c) What is the treatment of choice?

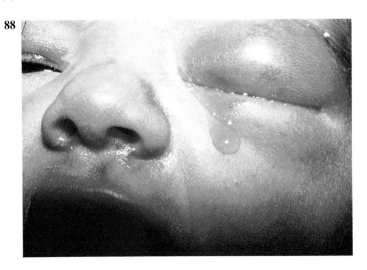

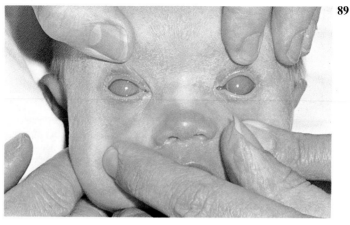

89 (a) What abnormality is shown?
   (b) What symptom is classical in such patients?
   (c) What treatment is required?

90 (a) What abnormalities does this child have?
(b) These findings are characteristic of which syndrome?
(c) Name one other syndrome in which similar features may be present?

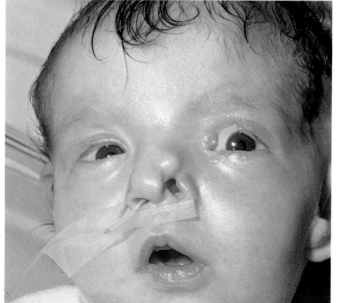

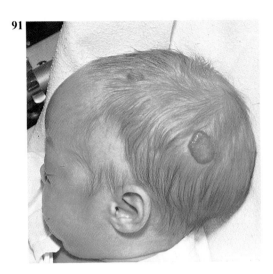

91 (a) What condition is shown?
(b) In what circumstances may surgical removal of the lesion be indicated?

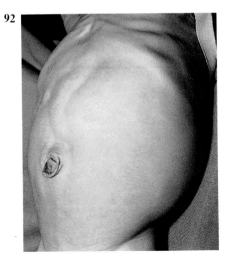

92 A five-week-old infant presented with a three-day history of vomiting. The vomitus was not bile-stained. The infant was constipated.
(a) What abnormality is seen in this illustration which was taken at the time of a test feed?
(b) What is the likely diagnosis?
(c) What abnormality of acid-base balance may be found and how should it be treated?

93 An asymptomatic newborn baby has a chubby leg.
(a) Is it abnormal?
(b) If so, why and with what condition may it be associated?

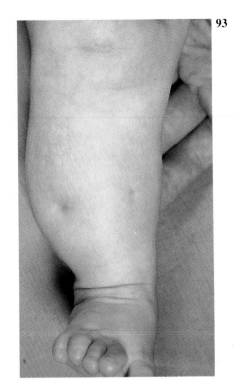

94 (a) What is wrong with this baby's umbilicus?
(b) What is the cause?

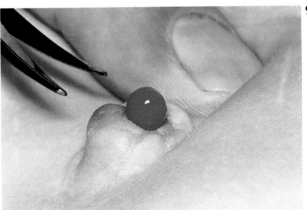

95

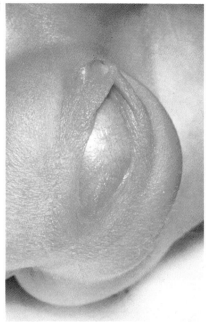

95 (a) What abnormality is apparent in the perineum of a newborn female infant?
(b) What is a common clinical presentation of this condition?
(c) What is the treatment of choice?

96

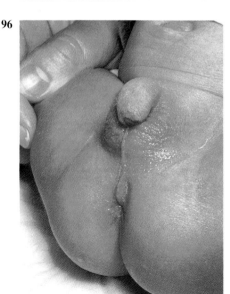

96 This baby was born at term to a healthy mother. Chromosomal examination was 46 XX. The serum 17 alpha hydroxyprogesterone level was markedly raised.
(a) What is the diagnosis?
(b) What is the mode of inheritance?
(c) What percentage of such children will be predisposed to electrolyte abnormalities?

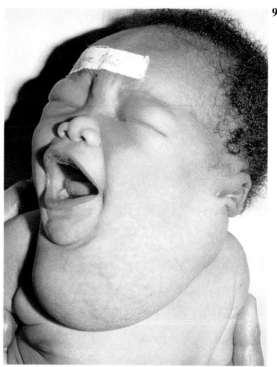

97 (a) What abnormality is demonstrated by this baby?
(b) What side effects may occur shortly after birth?

98 (a) What abnormality is seen in this infant's eyes?
(b) Of what disorder is the abnormality characteristic?

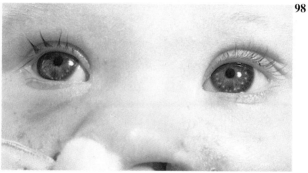

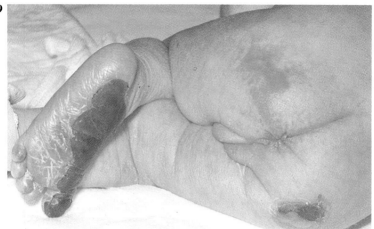

99 This premature infant had received neonatal intensive care and the lesions shown are iatrogenic.
(a) What procedure is likely to have been carried out?
(b) What is the pathogenesis of the lesions?

100 A 12-year-old presented with gradual loss of vision.
(a) What is the diagnosis?
(b) How is this condition usually inherited?

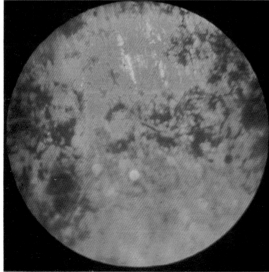

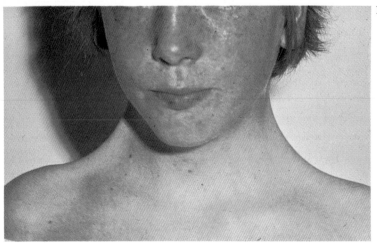

101 A seven-year-old girl was referred for a dermatological opinion. She had developed a facial rash in the previous six months. Apart from the rash, several café-au-lait spots were noted. Her past history revealed numerous convulsions and she was taking phenytoin.
(a) What is the diagnosis?
(b) Name two other skin manifestations of this condition.

102 A newborn infant attracted attention because of her feet.
(a) What is wrong?
(b) With what systemic abnormality is this sign characteristically associated?

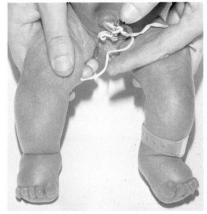

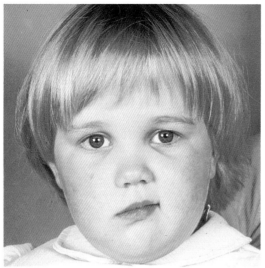

103 A two-year-old girl on antimitotic therapy for acute lymphoblastic leukaemia suddenly developed this lesion.
(a) What is the diagnosis?
(b) Name two possible aetiological factors.

104 (a) What physical signs are demonstrated in this knee?
(b) What is the likely underlying cause?

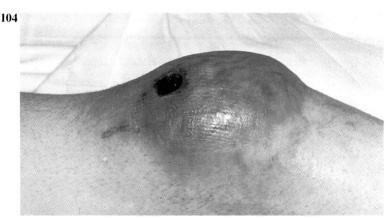

105 Describe four abnormalities shown in this peripheral blood film taken from a five-year-old West Indian boy.

106 A five-month-old boy presented with a dermatitis that had not responded to conventional topical treatment. On examination he had a similar eruption on the scalp and severe otitis externa. The liver was enlarged to 5cm and splenomegaly was present. A full blood count revealed a haemoglobin of 8g%, white cell count 1,200 with a differential of 60% neutrophils, 30% lymphocytes, 7% monocytes, 2% eosinophils, 1% basophils. The platelet count was 95,000 per cu.m.
(a) What is the likely diagnosis?
(b) How may this be proven most easily?

106

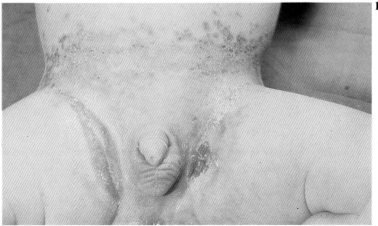

107

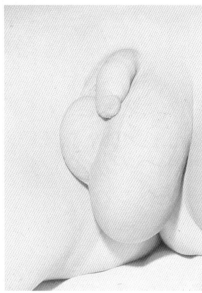

107 A five-year-old boy with anaemia, easy bruising and joint pain had this genital lesion. The scrotum did not transilluminate.

(a) What is the likely cause?

(b) What local treatment is necessary?

(c) How will local treatment influence prognosis?

108

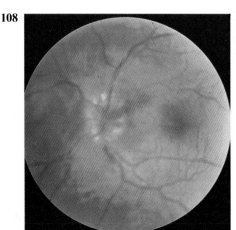

108 (a) Name three abnormalities seen in this fundus.

(b) Name four possible causes for these findings.

109 (a) Identify two abnormalities in this 11-year-old boy.
(b) What is the diagnosis?
(c) How is the condition inherited?

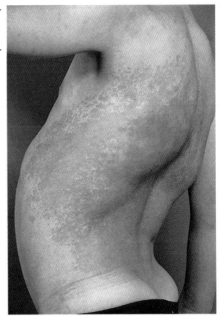

110 A two-year-old child was referred to an orthoptic clinic because of squint which had developed in the previous two weeks. Examination revealed paralysis of the right lateral rectus muscle.
(a) How should the child be managed?
(b) What underlying cause may account for this?

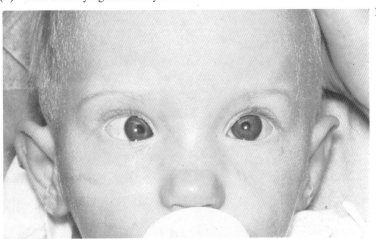

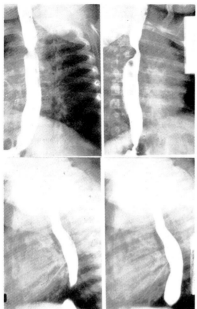

111 Radiographs demonstrate views obtained on a barium swallow examination performed on a child with recurrent vomiting and pneumonia.
(a) What is shown?
(b) What is the likely anomaly?

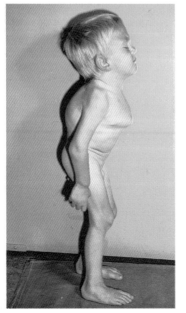

112 A six-year-old boy of normal intelligence has an inborn error of metabolism resulting in skeletal deformity.
(a) What is the diagnosis?
(b) What is the inheritance?
(c) What is the laboratory investigation of choice?

113 An 11-year-old girl with a three-month history of cough, weight loss and anorexia presented with leg lesions which had started two days previously.
(a) What is the nature of the skin lesion?
(b) What diagnosis must be considered in the light of this history and physical sign?

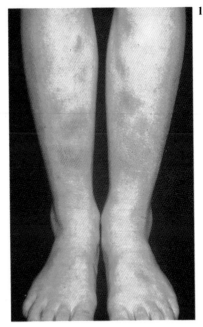

114 (a) What abnormality is shown?
(b) Name three syndromes in which this may occur.

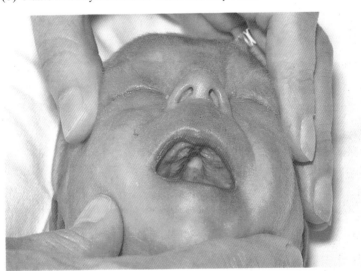

115 A larger than average seven-year-old girl is shown with a patient.

(a) Name three abnormalities visible in the patient.

(b) What is the possible diagnosis?

(c) What is the prognosis for final stature?

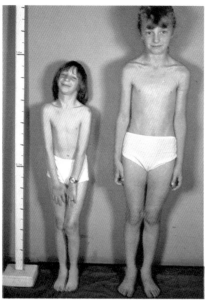

116 This is the postmortem appearance of an eleven-year-old child who had been slightly off-colour for one week. The family doctor had noted purulent tonsillitis and had prescribed penicillin. One afternoon after returning from swimming she felt faint and complained of shoulder pain. She became rapidly pale and shocked and was dead on arrival at the hospital.

(a) What was the immediate cause of death?

(b) What may have been the underlying illness?

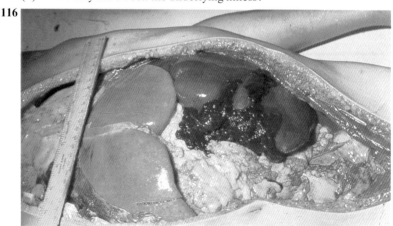

117 An 18-month-old child was born at 28 weeks' gestation and required prolonged neonatal intensive care.
(a) What abnormality is shown?
(b) What may have been the cause?

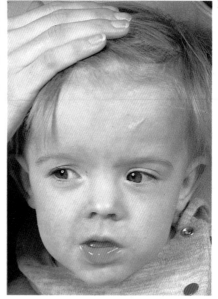

118 (a) What abnormality is seen in this newborn baby?
(b) What is the immediate danger?
(c) What other clinical problem may the infant encounter in the short term?
(d) What is the long term prognosis?

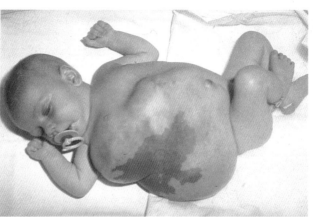

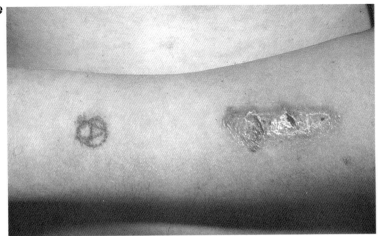

119 This is the forearm of a 14-year-old girl who has a disturbed family background.
(a) What lesions are shown?
(b) What is the likely cause of the inflamed lesion?

120 A seven-year-old boy was referred to Outpatients because of difficulty in micturition.
(a) What lesion is shown?
(b) What is the treatment?

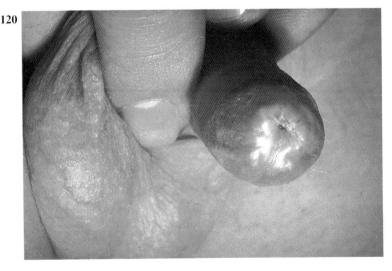

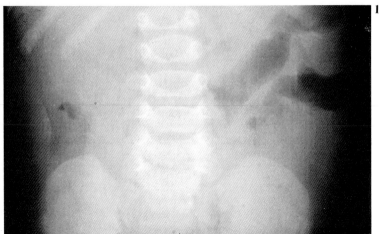

121 This is the plain abdominal radiograph of a three-year-old child who had been well until the previous day. Following an episode of diarrhoea she had intermittent attacks of abdominal pain and pallor. The general practitioner thought an abdominal mass was present but this was not confirmed by the casualty officer.
(a) What lesion is shown?
(b) What is the treatment of choice?
(c) What other modes of treatment are available?

122 (a) What physical condition can be seen in this three-year-old?
(b) Name four common causes.

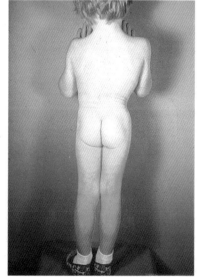

123

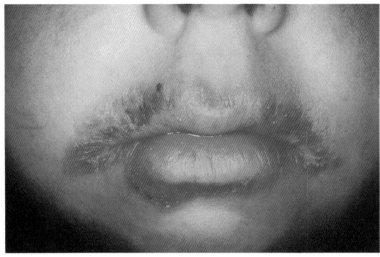

123 A four-year-old boy was noted to develop discoloration of his lips two months prior to acute admission to hospital with severe abdominal pain and melena. Similar lesions were noted on his mother's lips but she was asymptomatic.
(a) What is the diagnosis?
(b) What treatment is usually required?
(c) What is the main complication of this condition?

124

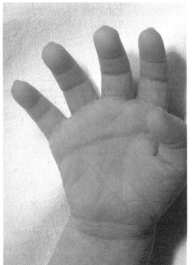

124 This is the hand of a one-year-old infant with developmental delay.
(a) Name two abnormalities.
(b) What is the likely diagnosis?
(c) What endocrine abnormality is more frequent in this syndrome?

125 An eight-year-old girl was referred because of short stature.
(a) What three abnormalities are seen?
(b) What is the diagnosis?
(c) How many children with this condition enter spontaneous puberty?

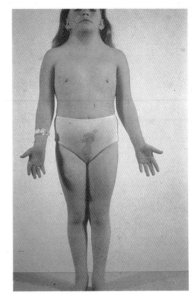

126 (a) What is apparent in this small intestinal wall?
(b) Name three possible causes.

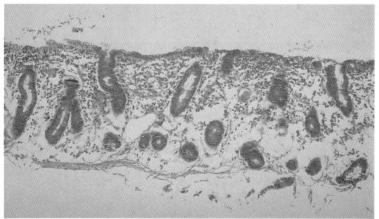

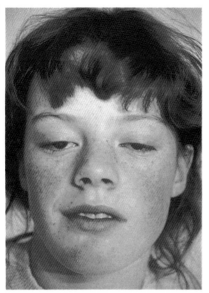

127 A 13-year-old girl presented to Outpatients with a six-months' history of muscle weakness which worsened as the day progressed. Her family doctor had thought she was suffering from hysteria. Referral was prompted by the development of diplopia.

(a) What physical sign is shown?

(b) What is the most likely diagnosis?

(c) How may this be confirmed?

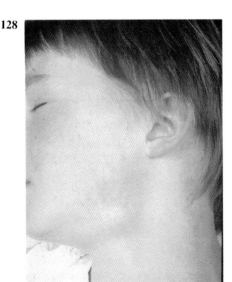

128 A four-year-old girl presented with pain on chewing.

(a) What abnormal physical sign is apparent?

(b) Name three possible causes.

129 A six-month-old infant was admitted to hospital for plastic surgery.
(a) What condition is shown?
(b) How is this inherited?

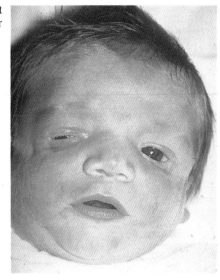

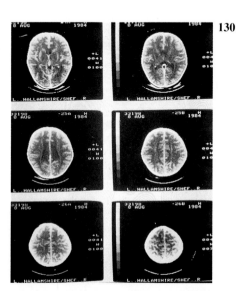

130 This is the CAT scan of a three-year-old admitted with blindness, cerebral palsy and macrocephaly.
(a) Describe the abnormalities seen in the scan.
(b) Suggest a possible pathophysiology and diagnosis.

131 (a) What is wrong with this boy?
(b) What is the mode of inheritance?

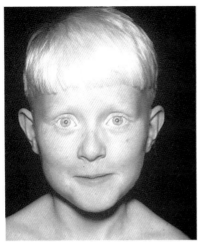

132 (a) What condition does this child have?
(b) What clinical feature does this have in common with osteogenesis imperfecta?
(c) Name two other common findings.

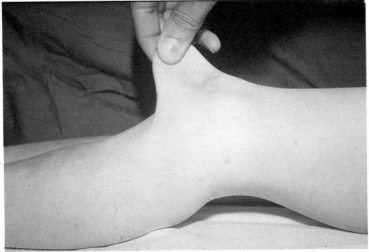

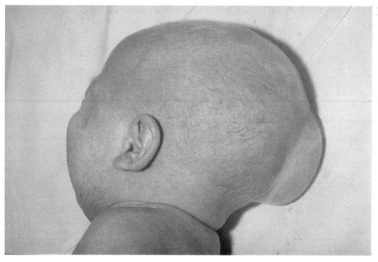

133 An eight-week-old infant presented with a lump on the head. Name three important differential diagnoses.

134 A three-year-old boy has severe bony deformities. His six-year-old brother is similarly affected.
(a) What is the diagnosis?
(b) How is this inherited?
(c) State another complication apart from bony deformities.

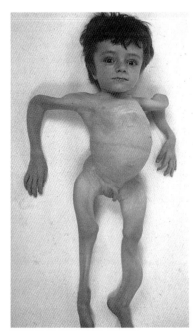

135

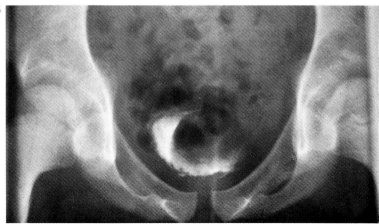

135 This radiograph was obtained during excretory urography of a six-year-old girl being investigated for recurrent urinary infection.
(a) What abnormality is shown?
(b) How is it caused?

136 This is the neck of a nine-year-old girl who presented in Dermatology outpatients. Her brother had been treated for a similar eruption two months earlier.
(a) What is the diagnosis?
(b) What is the aetiology?
(c) What is the prognosis without treatment?

136

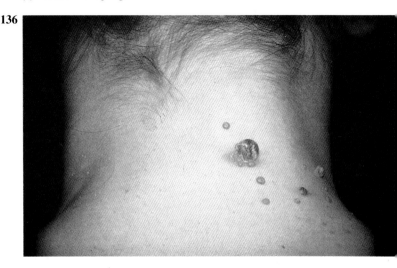

137 (a) What physical signs are demonstrated in this two-year-old girl?
(b) What is the diagnosis?
(c) What is the aetiological agent?

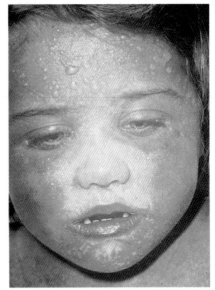

138 A three-year-old was admitted to hospital with a three-day history of diarrhoea, cough and general malaise. Examination revealed a fever of 38.5°C, general abdominal tenderness and 2cm splenomegaly. Twenty-four hours later he developed this rash.
(a) What is the diagnosis?
(b) Name three serious complications of the primary disease.

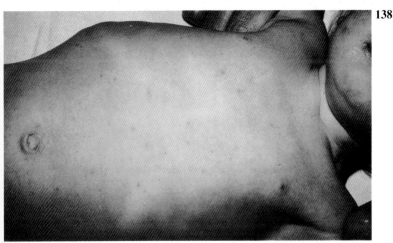

139 (a) What lesion is show
on this girl's face?
(b) What is the treatment c
choice?

140 A 10-year-old boy pre
sented to a mission hospita
with severe headache, back
ache and the above rash.
(a) What is the diagnosis?
(b) What abnormality i
characteristic in the white ce
count?
(c) What is the incubatio
period?

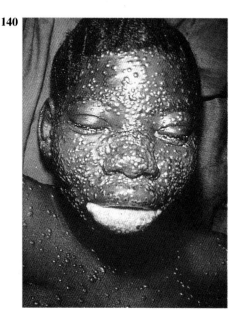

141 A twelve-year-old girl developed a very itchy rash on her hand two weeks previously. The lesions were spreading and now involved her forearm and chest.

(a) What is the diagnosis?

(b) What treatment is required?

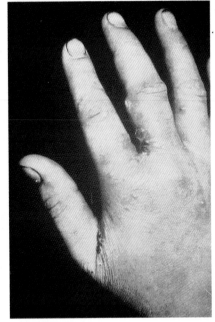

142 (a) What abnormality is shown in this 11-year-old girl?

(b) What is the likely diagnosis?

(c) What ocular complication may be found?

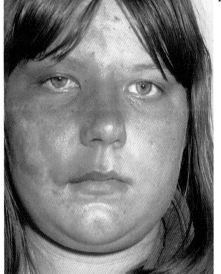

143

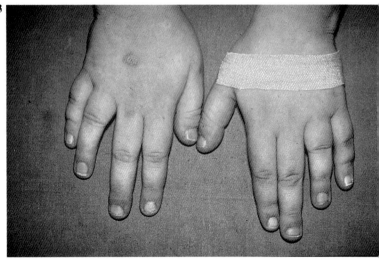

143 The hands of a five-year-old boy referred for assessment of growth failure and mental retardation.
(a) What abnormality is shown?
(b) What is the diagnosis?
(c) Name three other possible clinical findings.

144 A two-month-old infant was referred because of poor feeding. On examination he was noted to hold his head retracted and to have persistent flexion of the arms and legs. When questioned his mother said this had always been the case.
(a) What is the most likely diagnosis?
(b) Name three causes with origin in the neonatal period.

145 A three-year-old girl became ill one week previously when the only clinical abnormality was an abrasion on the cheek. This subsequently ulcerated with gradual development as shown, despite ampicillin treatment.
(a) What abnormality is seen?
(b) What is the likely causative organism?
(c) What is the treatment of choice?

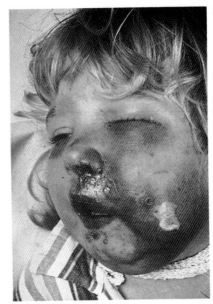

146 Radiograph of a 10-year-old boy who presented with shortness of breath which had become progressively worse over the preceding 48 hours.
(a) What abnormality is demonstrated?
(b) Name three possible causes.

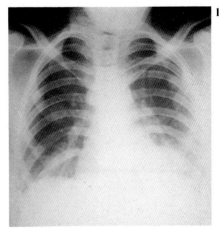

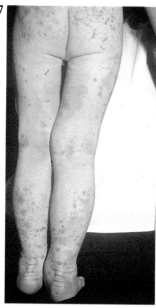

147 A five-year-old boy presented with abdominal pain and haematuria. The rash shown had developed 48 hours earlier.

(a) What is the diagnosis?

(b) What is the prognosis for the renal lesion?

(c) Name two causes for the abdominal pain.

148 (a) What is the cause of the lesion on this child's head?

(b) What is the pathogenesis?

(c) What is the treatment of choice?

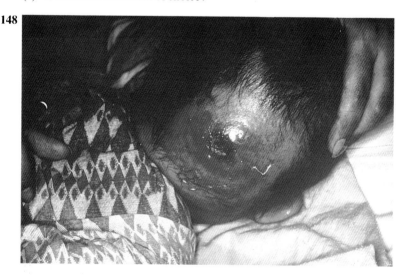

149 (a) What abnormality is present in this radiograph of a two-year-old?
(b) What is the most likely cause?

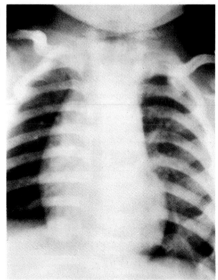

149

150 A three-year-old child presented to her family doctor with a history of proptosis, gradually worsening over the past three weeks. On examination a mass in the left flank was palpated.
(a) What is the diagnosis?
(b) Name three investigations that should be carried out.

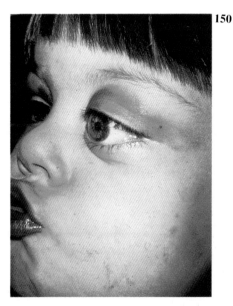

150

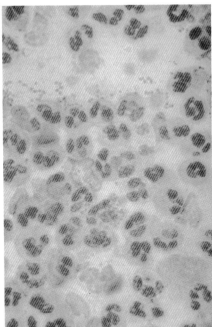

151 The microscopic appearance of CSF from a three-year-old child admitted with fever and neck stiffness.

(a) Name two abnormalities shown.

(b) What is the diagnosis?

(c) What is the treatment of choice?

152 Radiograph of a one-month-old infant who had received intensive care in the neonatal period.

(a) What abnormality is shown?

(b) What is the likely cause?

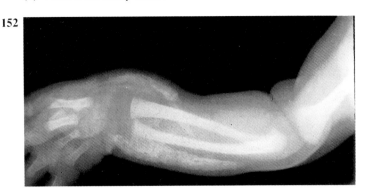

153 A 12-year-old girl was referred because of progressively deteriorating school performance.
(a) What abnormalities can be seen?
(b) What is the diagnosis?
(c) What is the treatment of choice?

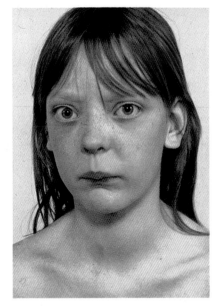

153

154 Radiograph of a four-year-old child with abdominal distension of three months' duration.
(a) What examination is being performed?
(b) What abnormality is demonstrated?
(c) What is the most likely cause?

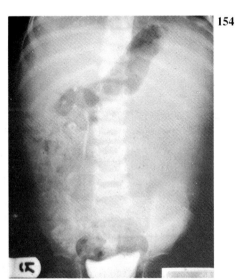

154

155

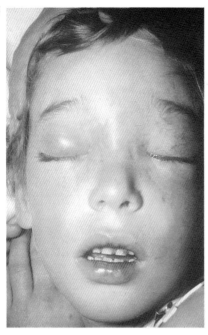

155 A five-year-old boy had a purulent nasal discharge for one week which had been treated with decongestants. The day before admission to hospital he developed a fever and drowsiness. He progressed rapidly to the appearance shown at the time of admission to hospital.
(a) What is the diagnosis?
(b) What is the treatment of choice?
(c) What may be revealed by examination of the CSF?

156

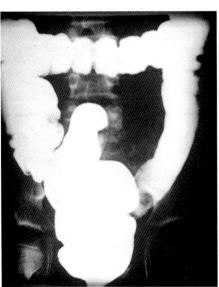

156 (a) Name two abnormalities seen in this radiograph of a barium enema examination.
(b) What is the diagnosis?
(c) Name the treatment of choice.

157 A three-year-old boy was referred because of recurrent fever and abnormal dentition. The fevers tended to occur most often during the summer and had been particularly troublesome during the family holiday in Spain. They had not responded to any form of therapy other than tepid sponging. On examination the teeth were noted to be widely spaced and peg-shaped.
(a) What is the diagnosis?
(b) What is the cause of the recurrent fevers?
(c) Name two further complications of this condition.

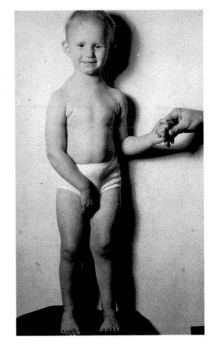

157

158 A four-year-old boy was referred because of developmental delay. Clinical examination revealed small nails, an ejection systolic murmur in the aortic area and a height and weight each below the 3rd centile. A radiograph of the wrist for the determination of bone age revealed increased bone density as a coincidental finding.
(a) What abnormalities can be seen?
(b) What is the diagnosis?
(c) What is the likely cause of his cardiac murmur?

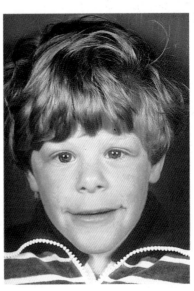

158

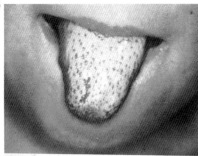

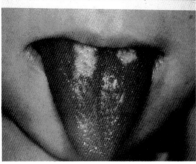

159 (a) What abnormalities are shown in these tongues?
(b) In what condition may they be seen?
(c) What is the treatment of choice for this condition?

160 A three-year-old girl was hospitalised because of a severe persistent cough.
(a) What abnormality is shown?
(b) What is the likely cause of her illness?

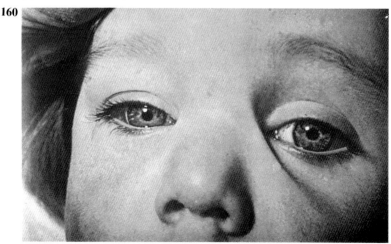

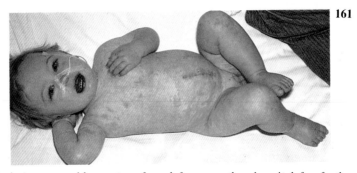

161 A two-year-old was transferred from another hospital for further investigation. She had been febrile, unwell and had generalised abdominal tenderness. Laparotomy revealed no abnormality. Two days later she developed this rash and generalised lymphadenopathy. On arrival at the referral centre, conjunctivitis, stomatitis and erythema of the hands and feet were also noted. Her fever continued to spike over the next week when peeling of the hands and feet occurred.
(a) What is the diagnosis?
(b) Name three further complications.
(c) What is the likely cause of her abdominal pain?

162 Specimen of brain and spinal cord taken from a short child who died suddenly, having been asymptomatic up to the moment of death.
(a) Describe the two abnormalities demonstrated.
(b) What was the child's likely primary pathology?

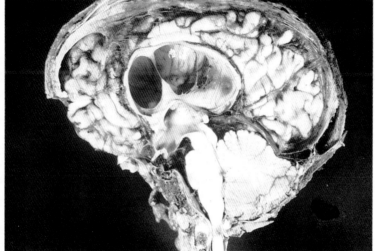

163

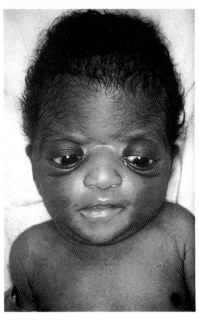

163 A two-year-old boy was referred to the Outpatient clinic because of his unusual appearance and failure to thrive. On examination he was noted to have broad thumbs and cryptorchidism.
(a) What abnormalities can be seen?
(b) What is the diagnosis?
(c) What is the prognosis for growth and for mental development?

164

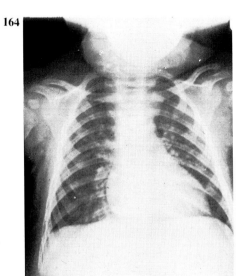

164 Radiograph of a five-year-old boy with a chronic cough that did not respond to repeated courses of antibiotics. His parents reported that he had fed well from birth but had gained weight slowly. Examination showed him to be below the 3rd centile for height and weight. Auscultation of the chest showed bilateral basal crepitations.
(a) What abnormality is seen in the radiograph?
(b) What is the most likely diagnosis?
(c) If the likely diagnosis is confirmed, what test should be carried out on his two-year-old sister?

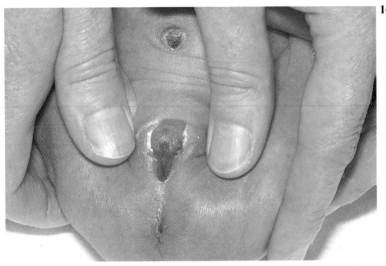

165 An eight-day-old infant was referred for assessment of ambiguous genitalia. There were no other clinical abnormalities. The chromosomes were 46 XY and the plasma 17–OH progesterone was normal. Careful examination of the inguinal canal revealed bilateral undescended gonads.
(a) What is the diagnosis?
(b) Name three investigations that may be helpful.

166 (a) What physical sign is shown in this two-year-old boy?
(b) State three possible hae-matological causes for this sign in his case.

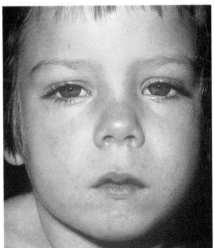

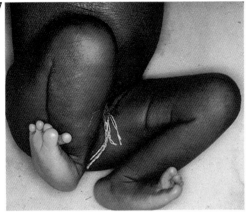

167 (a) What abnormality can be seen in this newborn baby?
(b) What is the anatomical defect?
(c) In what syndrome is this often found?

168 This operation was performed on a two-day-old infant who had been noted to have scrotal swelling, during the course of a routine examination.
(a) What is demonstrated?
(b) What additional surgical procedure is essential?

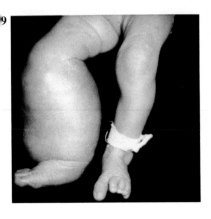

169 (a) What abnormality is shown?
(b) Name two important causes.

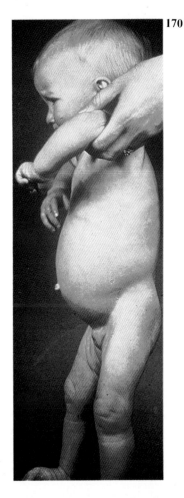

170 A 14-month-old child was referred to Outpatients because of irritability which had persisted from the age of three months. According to her parents she was anorexic and listless and prone to bouts of screaming. She showed no interest in play and disliked attention. On examination height and weight were below the 3rd centile; she appeared as shown.
(a) What abnormalities are demonstrated?
(b) What is the likely diagnosis?
(c) What is the investigation of choice?

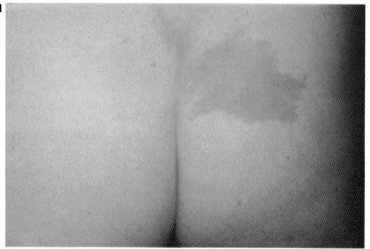

171 A two-year-old girl seen in Orthopaedic outpatients because of bowing of the legs, was referred to the medical Paediatric clinic because of early breast development. Additionally, the abnormal skin pigmentation shown was noted. A similar lesion was present on her neck.
(a) What is the diagnosis?
(b) How do these lesions differ from those seen in neurofibromatosis?

172 (a) What physical sign is demonstrated in this two-year-old?
(b) What is the most likely cause?
(c) State three reasons for this occurrence.

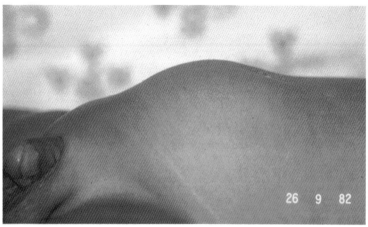

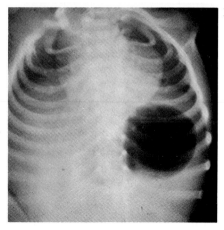

173 Radiograph of a one-day-old infant who had vomited all feeds.
(a) Name three abnormalities shown.
(b) What is the likely cause of the abnormalities?

174 (a) What condition is apparent?
(b) Name three pulmonary and three other causes.

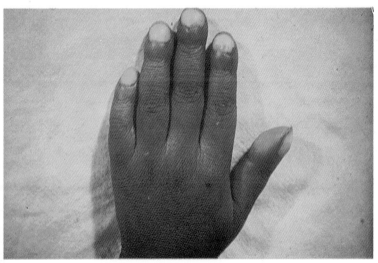

175

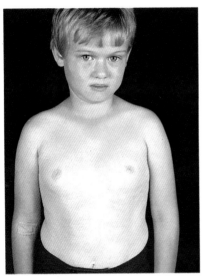

175 A seven-year-old boy was being teased at school.
(a) What is demonstrated?
(b) Name two possible causes.

176 The tongue of a 14-month-old child referred because of increasing hypotonia. Physical examination confirmed the hypotonia and demonstrated absent tendon reflexes and paradoxical breathing. Mental development was normal for his age.
(a) What is demonstrated?
(b) What is the most likely diagnosis?
(c) Which two investigations will help to confirm the diagnosis?

176

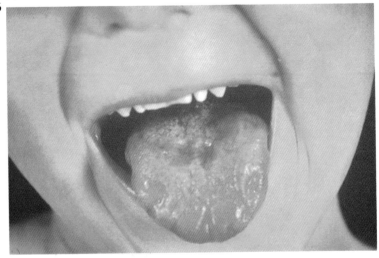

177 (a) What rash is shown?
(b) Name two conditions in which it may occur.

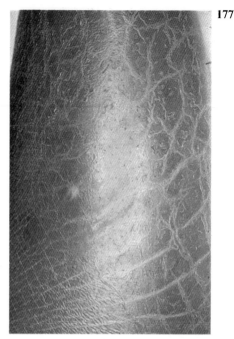

178 (a) What abnormality is demonstrated?
(b) Name three syndromes in which it may be found.

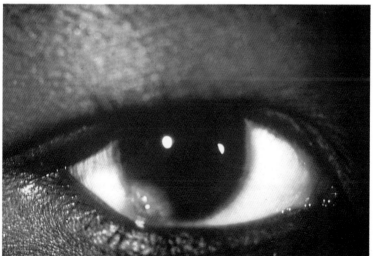

179

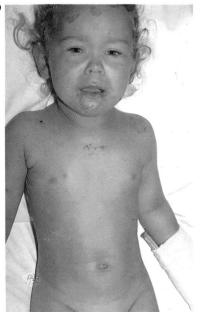

179 A three-year-old girl presented to her general practitioner with a pustule on the face. This was treated with topical antibiotics. Despite treatment the pustule increased in size before finally bursting. Three days later she developed a fever and erythema of the cheek which spread to the forehead and trunk. The rash then began to exfoliate and this coincided with increasing lethargy, anorexia and fever.

(a) What is the diagnosis?

(b) What is the aetiology of the rash?

(c) What treatment is indicated?

180 (a) What is this lesion?

(b) Name two ocular complications that may be seen.

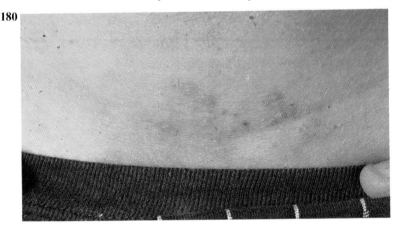

181 An 18-month-old infant presented with a swelling in the sacrococcygeal area of two months' duration. He had also lost weight and been anorexic with a cough. The swelling had increased in size gradually and the child had recently developed urinary retention. Laboratory investigations showed a raised alphafetoprotein and alpha 1 anti-trypsin in the blood.
(a) What is the diagnosis?
(b) What is the likely cause of the cough?

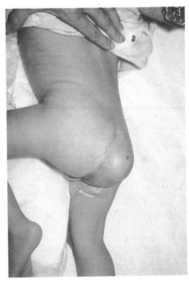

182 (a) What abnormality is shown?
(b) Name two syndromes in which this may occur.

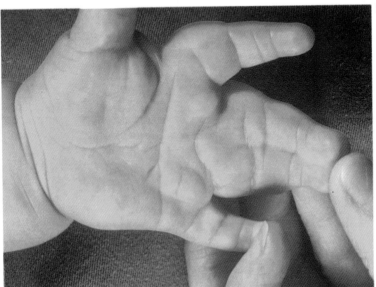

183 (a) What abnormality is shown?
(b) What is the aetiology?
(c) What treatment is available?

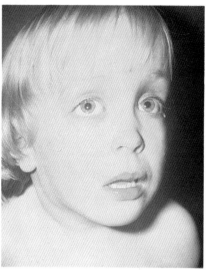

184 A 12-year-old boy was referred to a neurologist because of deteriorating school performance and increasing clumsiness. He also had the rash shown, moderate ataxia, hearing loss and retinal findings similar to those seen in retinitis pigmentosa. He deteriorated and six months later was unable to walk.
(a) Name the rash.
(b) What is the likely cause of the neurological deterioration?
(c) What treatment is available?

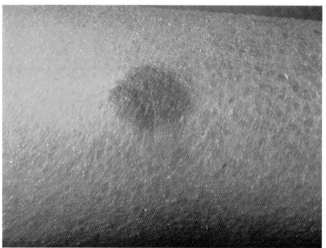

185 A rash was noted on a four-day-old baby.
(a) What is the most likely cause?
(b) What is the differential diagnosis?

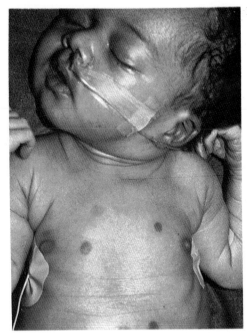

186 A four-year-old boy arrived at the Accident and Emergency Department three hours after having been stung by a wasp.
(a) What is the diagnosis?
(b) What is the treatment of choice?

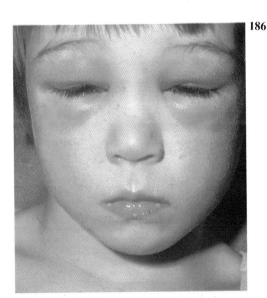

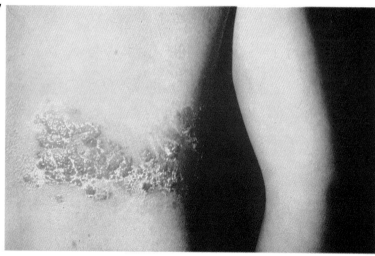

187 (a) What is this rash?
(b) What is the aetiology?
(c) How long does it take to resolve?

188 Radiograph of a two-year-old child of Asian parents who presented with a history of weight loss and cough.
(a) What abnormalities are shown?
(b) What is the likely diagnosis?
(c) What two investigations will be of benefit?

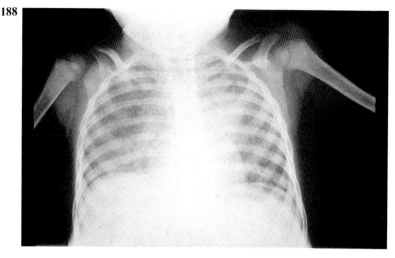

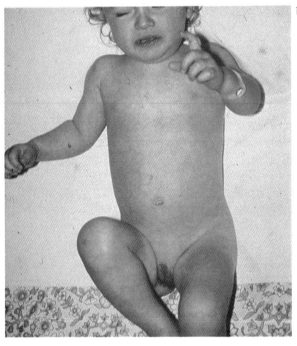

189 (a) What physical sign is apparent in this 18-month-old girl?
(b) Name three investigations of value in establishing the diagnosis.

190 (a) What physical sign is seen in this eight-year-old girl?
(b) Name two important causes.

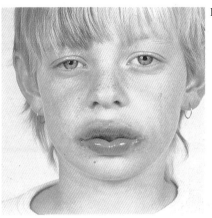

191

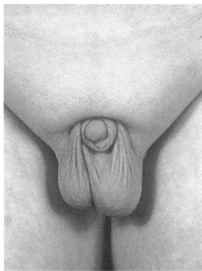

191 A nine-year-old boy presented to Outpatients because of school avoidance, particularly on days when he was due to have a P.E. lesson.
(a) What is the reason for his school phobia?
(b) State three possible causes.

192 A special investigation was performed on a two-year-old who presented with increasing weakness of the left leg.
(a) What investigation has been performed?
(b) What is demonstrated?
(c) What is the diagnosis?

192

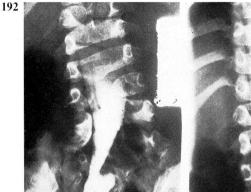
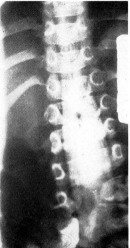

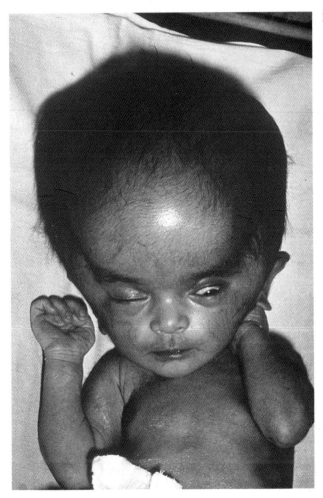

193 (a) What abnormal physical sign is demonstrated?
(b) What is the treatment of choice?
(c) Name five associated findings on examination.

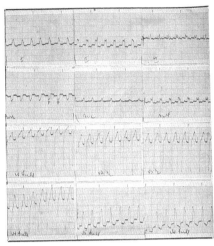

194 Cardiogram of a four-year-old presenting with shock and peripheral shutdown.
(a) What is demonstrated?
(b) What is the likely underlying cardiac lesion?

195 These lesions were noted on the scalp of a newborn baby.
(a) What are they?
(b) In which syndrome are they commonly found?
(c) What is the investigation of choice?

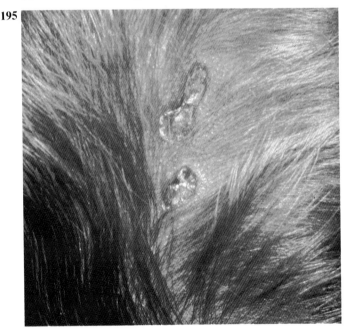

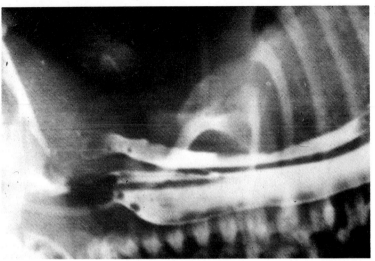

196 Radiograph shows a special investigation being performed on a three-month-old infant with recurrent wheeze.
(a) What is the investigation?
(b) What is demonstrated?
(c) What is the diagnosis?

197 A five-year-old boy presented to Outpatients with progressive difficulty in walking.
(a) What abnormalities are demonstrated?
(b) What is the diagnosis?
(c) What is the inheritance of this condition?

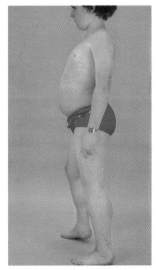

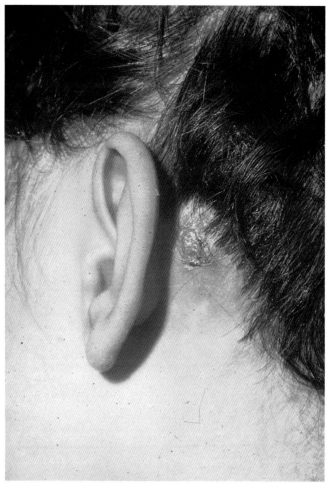

198 An 11-year-old boy presented to Outpatients with this lesion which had been present for eight months and discharging purulent material for six weeks. The lesion appeared after the boy had hurt himself in a swimming pool on holiday in the USA. Despite topical therapy the lesion had increased in size. A swab from the ulcer grew no bacteria after 48 hours but a 1:1000 Mantoux test produced a 7mm diameter reaction.
(a) What is the likely diagnosis?
(b) What is the treatment of choice?

199 A six-month-old infant was referred from a surgical clinic where he had been seen for repair of inguinal herniae. His length and weight had been noted incidentally to be below the 3rd centile, and his facial appearance had given cause for concern.

(a) What abnormalities are shown?

(b) What is the diagnosis?

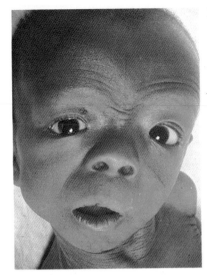

200 CAT scan of a five-month-old child who presented with convulsions, hypotonia and delayed motor milestones. What two abnormalities are present?

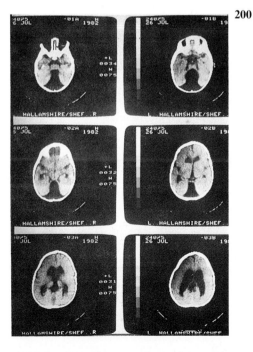

ANSWERS

1 (a) Erythema multiforme.
(b) The scalp.
(c) None – the rash is self-limiting.

2 Hypotonia at this age may be due to: Down's syndrome, birth asphyxia, hypothyroidism, prematurity, dystrophia myotonica, or maternal benzodiazepine administration.

3 (a) A pseudocyst of the pancreas.
(b) Following abdominal trauma.
(c) An abdominal mass.

4 (a) Juvenile myxoedema.
(b) Surprisingly, such patients are commonly said to have satisfactory school progress because of their placidity.
(c) Investigations of value include a serum thyroxin, TSH and a radiological determination of bone age.

5 (a) Chicken pox.
(b) Giant cells in scrapings from the lesion; virus culture; rise in antibody titre.

6 (a) Cystic kidneys. Note that it is not possible to distinguish between polycystic and multicystic kidneys on the radiograph.
(b) It is produced by drinking a fizzy liquid before the investigation, as an aid to visualisation of the kidneys.

7 (a) Russell–Silver dwarfism.
(b) Light-for-dates; short stature; hemihypotrophy.

8 (a) Von Willebrand's disease.
(b) Decreased Factor VIII concentration; decreased platelet adhesion; impaired platelet aggregation in the presence of ristocetin.

9 (a) Seborrhoeic dermatitis.
(b) Staphylococcus aureus or Candida albicans.
(c) The scalp.

10 (a) Herpangina.
(b) Coxsackie virus infection.
(c) Treatment is supportive, with particular attention to topical and systemic analgesia.

11 (a) Kwashiorkor.
(b) The post-weaning toddler.
(c) It is due to both fatty infiltration and oedema.

12 (a) A parotid abscess.
(b) Mumps.
(c) Staphylococcus aureus.

13 (a) The sex of the child – Hurler's syndrome is inherited as an autosomal recessive; Hunter's as an X-linked recessive.
(b) Nodules over the scapula are found in Hunter's but not in Hurler's syndrome.
(c) A cloudy cornea is found in Hurler's but not in Hunter's syndrome.

14 (a) Herpes stomatitis.
(b) Gentian violet has been applied topically.
(c) Application of topical acyclovir.

15 (a) Absence of secondary sexual characteristics; a short trunk and long legs.
(b) The most likely cause is anorexia nervosa but an endocrine diagnosis must be

considered. This could be primary gonadotrophin deficiency or gonadotrophin deficiency due to hypothalamo-pituitary disease.

16 (a) Crohn's disease.
(b) Stomatitis.
(c) Barium meal and follow-through.

17 (a) Diabetic lipoatrophy.
(b) Lipoatrophy (and hypertrophy) can be lessened by rotation of injection site and by the use of monocomponent insulin preparations.

18 (a) Achondroplasia.
(b) Inheritance is as an autosomal dominant.
(c) Kyphosis.

19 (a) Mumps.
(b) Displacement of the tonsils toward the midline.
(c) Further complications include pancreatitis and orchitis.

20 (a) Bow legs.
(b) No cause discoverable.
(c) Vitamin D deficient rickets.
(d) Renal rickets.

21 (a) Cri-du-chat syndrome.
(b) Hypertelorism and prominent ears.
(c) Adult height is reduced but longevity is unaffected.

22 (a) Measles.
(b) Complications include encephalitis, pneumonitis and subacute sclerosing panencephalitis.
(c) Other hospitalised patients in contact should be given protective immuno-globulin injections, if they are immunodeficient or under the age of nine months. Otherwise they should be vaccinated against measles immediately if this has not been done.

23 (a) Posterior urethral valves.
(b) This may present as an abdominal mass, dribbling of urine or a urinary tract infection.
(c) The micturating cystourethrogram should be performed suprapubically.

24 (a) Jaundice, a caput medusa and abdominal swelling with an umbilical hernia.
(b) Biliary atresia.
(c) Treatment is surgical and involves anastomosis of the duodenum to the porta hepatis.

25 (a) A protruding tongue.
(b) Down's syndrome, hypothyroidism and the Beckwith–Wiedemann syndrome.

26 (a) Mediastinal shift, a hyperexpanded left lung and consolidation in the right middle and lower lobes.
(b) These findings together with the history are compatible with the aspiration of a foreign body.

27 (a) A white membrane on the tonsils.
(b) Infection with Group A streptococcus, diphtheria, Epstein–Barr virus or adenovirus.

28 (a) Dactylitis.
(b) This is commonly caused by juvenile rheumatoid arthritis or by sickle cell disease.

29 (a) Stevens–Johnson syndrome.
(b) Mycoplasma pneumoniae.

30 (a) Staining of the teeth.

(b) The two commonest causes are hyperbilirubinaemia in the neonatal period and tetracycline treatment.

(c) Eight years, although hyperbilirubinaemia may affect the first permanent molars.

31 (a) Monilial paronychia.

(b) Oral griseofulvin with the option of a topical antifungal agent.

32 (a) Hyperplasia of the gums.

(b) Causes include phenytoin administration, scurvy, and infiltration, eg sarcoidosis or Crohn's disease.

33 (a) An ampicillin rash.

(b) Infectious mononucleosis (glandular fever).

(c) Monospot test; abnormal lymphocytes in the peripheral blood smear.

34 (a) Marasmus.

(b) The basal metabolic rate may be reduced and the core temperature may be low.

(c) The older child will no longer receive breast milk.

35 (a) Lipohypertrophy associated with the site of insulin injection.

(b) His overall management could be adversely affected if he persists in giving his injections into those sites since this may result in irregular insulin absorption and poor metabolic control.

36 (a) The child is hypothyroid.

(b) A serum TSH level is likely to be pathologically raised.

(c) A wrist radiograph is likely to show a delay in the appearance of the carpal bones and epiphyses.

37 (a) An intraspinal mass displacing the sacrum.

(b) An enlarged bladder.

(c) An intraspinal tumour, probably a sacral lipoma or dermoid.

38 (a) Patau's syndrome; this is due to trisomy 13.

(b) The feet are often rockerbottom in shape.

(c) The long term prognosis is poor; the patients usually die before the age of one year.

39 (a) Precocious true breast development.

(b) Premature thelarche.

(c) Determination of the bone age, the serum oestrogen concentration, abdominal ultrasound searching for ovarian pathology, and gonadotrophin measurement in response to LHRH stimulation.

40 (a) Nephrotic syndrome.

(b) Approximately 70 per cent.

(c) Glucocorticoids.

41 (a) Wilson's disease.

(b) Penicillamine.

(c) Inheritance is autosomal recessive.

42 (a) Skin necrosis and sloughing due to disseminated intravascular coagulation.

(b) Meningococcal septicaemia.

43 (a) Atrophy of the subcutaneous tissue, particularly of the upper arms and legs.

(b) Partial lipodystrophy.

44 (a) Hiatus hernia.

(b) Failure to thrive; recurrent chest infections; anaemia.

45 (a) Inflammation of the perineal region accompanied by a fistula.
(b) Crohn's disease.
(c) A barium meal and follow-through examination.

46 (a) 'Railroad' calcification of the cerebral blood vessels due to Sturge–Weber syndrome.
(b) Inheritance is sporadic.

47 (a) She is tall and has long arms and legs.
(b) Marfan's syndrome and homocystinuria.
(c) Marfan's syndrome is inherited dominantly whereas homocystinuria is a recessive condition.

48 (a) Low set ears.
(b) Down's, Edward's, Patau's, Potter's syndromes.

49 (a) Tall stature, enlarged penis.
(b) True precocious puberty, adrenogenital syndrome, hypothalamic tumour.

50 (a) Diphtheria.
(b) Systemic penicillin and antitoxin are urgently required.
(c) Bacteriological examination of a throat swab taken after removal of the tonsillular exudate and a fluorescent antibody test.

51 (a) Tuberculous cervical lymphadenopathy.
(b) Mantoux test and excision biopsy of the swelling.

52 (a) Colloid goitre.
(b) Confirmation that the swelling is due to thyroid enlargement is made by palpation from behind and upward movement of the gland on swallowing.
(c) Thyroxine in endemic areas.

53 (a) Infected thyroglossal cyst.
(b) Antibiotic therapy initially, followed by excision of the cyst.

54 (a) The baby has the characteristic facies of Crouzon's disease.
(b) Premature fusion of the basal sutures.

55 (a) Ataxia telangiectasia.
(b) Inheritance is autosomal recessive.
(c) Increased frequency of infection due to immunological deficiency; increased incidence of brain tumours.

56 (a) Cigarette burn. This should be suspected because of the circular nature of the lesion and its location.
(b) When non-accidental injury is suspected a skeletal survey and clotting screen is usually carried out if bruising is present.

57 (a) Prune belly syndrome.
(b) Urinary tract abnormalities and constipation.

58 (a) Sarcoma botryoides due to a rhabdomyosarcoma of the vagina.
(b) Infants of less than one year.
(c) Surgery and radiotherapy.

59 (a) Meconium is being passed per urethrum.
(b) A rectourethral fistula complicating anorectal agenesis.
(c) Poor.

60 (a) Marked abdominal distension.
(b) Hirschsprung's disease.
(c) Treatment will probably involve a colostomy followed by resection of the affected segment and a pull-through operation.

61 (a) A cataract.
(b) A cataract found at the age of one month could be due to Down's syndrome, galactosaemia or congenital rubella.

62 (a) Multiple fistulae of Crohn's disease resulting in complete necrosis of the abdominal wall.
(b) In her immediate management it is important to ensure adequate nutrition which can be best given parenterally. In the long term, intestinal resection may be necessary.

63 (a) The pathological specimen shows corrosive oesophagitis.
(b) This is most commonly the result of accidental ingestion of a corrosive substance such as caustic soda (lye).

64 (a) Unilateral gynaecomastia.
(b) Treatment is conservative.
(c) Gynaecomastia may arise also as a complication of drug therapy or rarely due to oestrogen secreting tumours.

65 (a) Pectus excavatum.
(b) It is congenital in origin.
(c) The scapula.

66 (a) A rectal prolapse.
(b) This should alert the clinician to consider cystic fibrosis.
(c) Treatment is by gentle manual replacement if this does not occur spontaneously.

67 (a) Balanoposthitis due to inflammation of the glans and foreskin of the penis extending into the shaft.
(b) Antibiotics followed in some cases by the separation of adhesions.

68 (a) Spinal dermoid cyst which, in this case, had communicated through a defect in the vertebral arch to the spinal theca.
(b) An emergency myelogram.

69 (a) Coarse, mop-like hair; eyebrows that meet in the midline; a large upper lip; micrognathia and short, pointed extremities of the limbs.
(b) Cornelia de Lange syndrome.
(c) The prognosis is poor: the infants subsequently show growth failure and severe mental retardation.

70 (a) Knock knees or genu valgum.
(b) Under five years old.
(c) A greenstick fracture of the femur.

71 (a) Genu recurvatum which results from posterior dislocation of the knees.
(b) Genu recurvatum may be congenital, secondary to cerebral palsy, osteomyelitis or poliomyelitis.

72 (a) Sprengel's deformity.
(b) Failure of descent of the scapula from the neck resulting in elevation of the shoulder on the affected side.
(c) There may be limitation of abduction of the arm and associated rib and vertebral anomalies.

73 (a) Lobster-claw hand.
(b) It is seen in Cornelia de Lange syndrome.
(c) Cleft lip and palate.

74 (a) Burkitt's lymphoma.
(b) The Epstein–Barr virus.
(c) The swelling also may be caused by an adamantinoma.

75 (a) Gross abdominal distension associated with widespread erythema of the anterior abdominal wall.
(b) Necrotising enterocolitis, volvulus, primary peritonitis, or spontaneous perforation of the bowel.

76 (a) Cushing's syndrome.
(b) If untreated, this will result in stunting of final adult height.
(c) It is most likely to be due to a pituitary tumour.

77 (a) The child has an imperforate anus. She has passed meconium through a rectovaginal fistula. In the illustration, the upper opening is the urethra and the lower a common orifice for the vagina and rectum.
(b) A defunctioning colostomy followed by reconstruction of a functioning anus.

78 (a) There is hemihypotrophy, the left side of the face being larger than the right.
(b) Wilms' tumour.

79 (a) Hydrops fetalis.
(b) Renal aplasia, congenital infection, achondroplasia, congenital nephrotic syndrome, but many are idiopathic.

80 (a) The twins are classical examples of the twin-to-twin transfusion syndrome due to an arteriovenous fistula in a common placenta.
(b) The polycythaemic infant.
(c) A modified partial exchange transfusion in which blood is removed and replaced by plasma.

81 (a) Beckwith–Wiedemann syndrome.
(b) There may be a horizontal crease in the ear lobe.
(c) They may suffer hypoglycaemic crises.

82 The lesion could be a nasal encephalocele, a nasal dermoid, or a cavernous haemangioma.

83 (a) The infant has no nose, bilateral cleft lip and hypotelorism.
(b) Holoprosencephaly.
(c) There may be fusion of the lateral ventricles.
(d) Chromosomal examination may reveal trisomy 13.

84 (a) A subdural effusion.
(b) This could have occurred as a result of trauma during or after birth or as a result of meningitis.

85 (a) A large bilateral intraventricular haemorrhage.
(b) Hypercapnea, prematurity and respiratory distress.
(c) Mental handicap, cerebral palsy and hydrocephalus.

86 (a) Sternomastoid tumour.
(b) Leave it alone.
(c) They mostly occur following uncomplicated delivery.

87 (a) Complete left facial palsy.
(b) This is usually due to pressure on the facial nerve during forceps delivery. The prognosis for spontaneous recovery is good.

88 (a) Conjunctivitis.
(b) This may be gonococcal in aetiology, but can be due to chlamydiae or other bacteria.
(c) Systemic antibiotics.

89 (a) Congenital glaucoma.
(b) Photophobia.
(c) Surgery is urgently required.

90 (a) A coloboma of the left upper eyelid and the left nostril.
(b) The condition is named Goldenhar's syndrome.
(c) Patau's syndrome.

91 (a) A cavernous haemangioma of the scalp.
(b) Surgical removal is rarely indicated. If the haemangioma is causing trouble due to bleeding or platelet consumption, surgical treatment by embolisation or thrombosis is preferable.

92 (a) Waves of peristalsis in the epigastrium.
(b) Pyloric stenosis.
(c) The baby is likely to have a metabolic alkalosis and should be treated with intravenous saline and potassium supplements.

93 (a) The abnormality is a dimple over the tibia and fibula.
(b) It is characteristic of hypophosphatasia, a rare condition due to deficiency of alkaline phosphatase which results in failure of calcification of all bones.

94 (a) An umbilical polyp.
(b) This arises when the vitelline duct fails to obliterate and atrophy.

95 (a) Hydrocolpos resulting from retention of uterine and vaginal secretions due to an imperforate hymen.
(b) An abdominal mass.
(c) Incision of the hymen.

96 (a) Congenital adrenal hyperplasia, in this case due to 21-hydroxylase deficiency.
(b) Inheritance is autosomal recessive.
(c) Approximately 30 per cent of such patients will have salt-losing crises.

97 (a) A cystic hygroma of the neck, not a goitre.
(b) The lesion may cause pressure symptoms on the trachea.

98 (a) Brushfield spots.
(b) Down's syndrome.

99 (a) Umbilical arterial catheterisation.
(b) The skin necrosis of the right buttock and left foot may be embolic or may follow spasm and thrombosis of the internal obturator artery and femoral artery.

100 (a) Retinitis pigmentosa.
(b) As an autosomal recessive, autosomal dominant or X-linked recessive. The most common inheritance is autosomal recessive.

101 (a) Adenoma sebaceum.
(b) Shagreen patches; periungual fibroma; hypopigmented macules.

102 (a) Lymphoedema of the feet and legs.
(b) This is a classical sign of Turner's syndrome.

103 (a) Seventh nerve palsy.
(b) Meningeal infiltration by leukaemic cells, a bleed into the central nervous system due to thrombocytopenia, neuropathy associated with vincristine therapy.

104 (a) Haemarthrosis of the knee.
(b) This is most likely to be due to Factor VIII deficiency or haemophilia.

105 The film is typical of sickle cell disease. In it are seen sickle cells, target cells, anisocytosis and hypochromia.

106 (a) Histiocytosis X.
(b) By histological examination of a skin biopsy.

107 (a) Leukaemic infiltration of the testis.
(b) Irradiation.
(c) This has no effect on the overall prognosis.

108 (a) Blurring of the optic disc, fundal haemorrhage and tortuosity of the vessels.
(b) Hypertension, intracranial neoplasm, intracranial haemorrhage, meningitis, or other causes of raised intracranial pressure.

109 (a) A large neurofibroma and lordo-scoliosis.
(b) Neurofibromatosis.
(c) Inheritance is autosomal dominant.

110 (a) Acute onset paralysis of any external ocular muscle requires vigorous investigation for the cause.
(b) Examples of lesions resulting in external rectus paralysis are: intracranial tumour, neurodegenerative disorders.

111 (a) Indenting of the oesophagus due to extramural pressure.
(b) A vascular ring.

112 (a) Morquio's syndrome.
(b) Autosomal recessive.
(c) A key investigation is examination of the urine for keratan and chondroitin sulphate.

113 (a) Erythema nodosum.
(b) This is associated with a number of diagnoses but in this case tuberculosis must be considered seriously.

114 (a) A cleft of the soft and hard palate not associated with hare lip.
(b) Pierre Robin, Patau's, Opitz, orocraniodigital syndromes.

115 (a) Microcephaly, a large nose and shortness.
(b) Seckel's bird-headed dwarfism.
(c) Adult height is markedly reduced in those who survive.

116 (a) Splenic rupture.
(b) This may have occurred as a complication of infectious mononucleosis.

117 (a) Scar on the forehead.
(b) This was due to a drip which had tissued.

118 (a) A huge thoracoabdominal cavernous haemangioma.
(b) It might rupture.
(c) Bleeding from other sites due to thrombocytopenia as a result of platelets being consumed within the cavernous haemangioma.
(d) The long term prognosis is good, the haemangioma will gradually regress and fade.

119 (a) A self-inflicted tattoo and dermatitis artefacta.
(b) The girl scraping the skin on her arm.

120 (a) He is suffering from phimosis.
(b) Circumcision.

121 (a) Intussusception.
(b) Hydrostatic reduction.
(c) Surgical excision may be required.

122 (a) Scoliosis.
(b) It may be congenital, due to spina bifida, neurofibromatosis, or other spinal destructive lesions such as tuberculosis.

123 (a) Peutz–Jeghers' syndrome.
(b) Supportive.
(c) Malignant change of the bowel polyps.

124 (a) The hand is spade-shaped and shows a single palmar crease and brachydactyly.
(b) Down's syndrome.
(c) Hypothyroidism is more common than in the general population.

125 (a) Webbing of the neck, hypertelorism, increased carrying angle of the arms and widely spaced nipples.
(b) Turner's syndrome.
(c) Approximately 10 per cent.

126 (a) Villous atrophy.
(b) Coeliac disease, tropical sprue, cow's milk protein intolerance, giardiasis, iron deficiency.

127 (a) Ptosis.
(b) Myasthenia gravis.
(c) By reversal of the abnormal clinical signs by intravenous administration of edrophonium chloride.

128 (a) A swelling in the submandibular region.
(b) A dental abscess, lymphadenitis or, as was the case in this patient, inflammation and enlargement of the submandibular gland.

129 (a) Treacher–Collins syndrome.
(b) Inheritance is autosomal dominant.

130 (a) Cerebral atrophy, derangement and vacuolisation of the white matter.
(b) This is due to spongy degeneration of the white matter, in this case the result of Canavan's disease.

131 (a) He is an albino.
(b) Autosomal recessive.

132 (a) Ehlers Danlos syndrome.
(b) Blue sclerae are found in both.
(c) Easy bruising and subcutaneous calcification.

133 The lump could be due to a haematoma, abscess or an encephalocoele. An encephalocoele is usually mid-line; the lump appears to be slightly lateral to the mid-line, making this diagnosis less likely.

134 (a) Osteogenesis imperfecta.
(b) Autosomal dominant.
(c) Deafness.

135 (a) A ureterocele.
(b) Ureteric obstruction with consequent ballooning of the distal ureter as it enters the bladder.

136 (a) Molluscum contagiosum.
(b) Infection with a DNA virus of the pox group.
(c) The condition is eventually self-limiting.

137 (a) A red desquamating rash with circumoral pallor.
(b) Scarlet fever.
(c) An erythrogenic toxin from Group A Streptococcal infection.

138 (a) Typhoid fever.
(b) Encephalopathy, intestinal perforation and pneumonia.

139 (a) Tinea corporis.
(b) Topical antifungal agents with possible oral griseofulvin.

140 (a) Smallpox.
(b) Neutropenia.
(c) Twelve days.

141 (a) Scabies.
(b) Topical benzyl benzoate or gamma benzene hexachloride. Eradication involves treatment of the rest of the family and careful cleaning of clothes and bed linen.

142 (a) A haemangioma over the maxillary branch of trigeminal nerve.
(b) Sturge–Weber syndrome.
(c) The development of glaucoma.

143 (a) Shortening of the fourth and fifth metacarpals.
(b) This is a characteristic finding in pseudohypoparathyroidism.
(c) Subcutaneous calcification, bowing of the legs, cataracts, thickening of the skull.

144 (a) Cerebral palsy.
(b) Perinatal asphyxia, hypoglycaemia or meningitis.

145 (a) Facial cellulitis.
(b) Staphylococcal infection.
(c) Parenteral flucloxacillin and fusidic acid.

146 (a) A left pleural effusion.
(b) Bacterial pneumonia, tuberculosis or malignancy.

147 (a) Henoch–Schönlein purpura.
(b) In the majority of cases there is complete recovery.
(c) Inflammation of the bowel wall associated with gastrointestinal haemorrhage, or intussusception.

148 (a) Anthrax.
(b) Contact with an animal product containing spores of the anthrax bacillus.
(c) Penicillin.

149 (a) Healing fracture of the posterior aspect of the ninth right rib.
(b) This finding immediately suggests non-accidental injury.

150 (a) The child has a retro-orbital metastasis of tumour, most probably a neuroblastoma.
(b) Ultrasound examination of the abdomen, whole body CAT scan and biopsy of the mass.

151 (a) Numerous pus cells with intracellular and extracellular Gram negative diplococci.
(b) Meningococcal meningitis.
(c) Intravenous penicillin.

152 (a) Subcutaneous calcification.
(b) This was a complication arising from subcutaneous leakage of calcium being given intravenously.

153 (a) A goitre and proptosis.
(b) Thyrotoxicosis.
(c) Carbimazole.

154 (a) Intravenous pyelogram.
(b) The left kidney is non-functioning; there is displacement of the stomach to the right.
(c) Wilms' tumour.

155 (a) Cavernous sinus thrombosis.
(b) Urgent surgical treatment.
(c) Raised pressure, an increase in both the red and white cell count and an elevated protein concentration.

156 (a) Loss of the normal haustrations, and generalised narrowing of the ascending and transverse colon.
(b) Ulcerative colitis.
(c) Initial therapy would include corticosteroids and salazopyrine.

157 (a) Anhydrotic ectodermal dysplasia.
(b) Absence of sweat glands.
(c) Recurrent pulmonary infections, atrophic rhinitis, dysphonia.

158 (a) Anteverted nostrils and an elfin facies.
(b) Idiopathic hypercalcaemia.
(c) Supravalvular aortic stenosis.

159 (a) White and red strawberry tongue.
(b) Scarlet fever.
(c) Penicillin.

160 (a) Subconjunctival haemorrhage.
(b) Bordetella pertussis.

161 (a) Kawasaki disease (Mucocutaneous lymph node syndrome).
(b) Encephalitis, arthritis, proteinuria, and arterial aneurysms, particularly affecting the coronary artery.
(c) Mesenteric adenitis.

162 (a) Hydrocephalus and compression of the cervical cord.
(b) Achondroplasia.

163 (a) A prominent forehead, marked epicanthic folds and downward slanting eyes.
(b) Rubinstein–Taybi syndrome.
(c) Somatic growth is poor and most affected patients are mentally handicapped.

164 (a) Numerous areas of patchy consolidation with bronchial wall thickening.
(b) Cystic fibrosis.
(c) A sweat test.

165 (a) Intersex.
(b) Rectal examination for palpation of the cervix, laparoscopy and/or pelvic ultrasound to identify the internal genitalia, and gonadal biopsy to determine whether or not one or both gonads is an ovotestis.

166 (a) He is jaundiced.
(b) Spherocytosis, elliptocytosis, thalassemia major, autoimmune haemolytic anaemia, G6PD deficiency or PK deficiency.

167 (a) Rockerbottom feet.
(b) A vertical talus.
(c) Edward's syndrome.

168 (a) Torsion of the testis.
(b) The other testis should be operated on also to prevent the occurrence of torsion.

169 (a) Elephantiasis.
(b) The massive swelling of the leg was caused in this patient by a hamartomatous malformation of blood vessels, lymphatics and subcutaneous tissue. It may also be caused by filariasis.

170 (a) Abdominal distention associated with wasting of the limbs.
(b) Coeliac disease.
(c) A jejunal biopsy and treatment with gluten exclusion.

171 (a) McCune–Albright syndrome (Polyostotic fibrous dysplasia).
(b) The café-au-lait spot in McCune–Albright syndrome has characteristic ragged edges, compared to the smooth edged lesions seen in neurofibromatosis.

172 (a) A suprapubic swelling.
(b) Bladder enlargement.
(c) Following outlet obstruction due to tumour, spinal injury or shock. It may occur also in hyponatraemia.

173 (a) Gastric distention, splaying of the ribs, abdominal distention and no air in the abdomen distal to the stomach.
(b) Complete pyloric obstruction.

174 (a) Clubbing.
(b) Cystic fibrosis, lung abscess or bronchiectasis. It may complicate cardiac conditions such as truncus arteriosus or Fallot's tetralogy; it is seen also in cirrhosis of the liver.

175 (a) Pathological gynaecomastia.
(b) Precocious puberty or an oestrogen secreting tumour.

176 (a) Fibrillation of the tongue.
(b) Werdnig–Hoffman disease.
(c) An EMG and muscle biopsy.

177 (a) 'Crazy paving' dermatitis.
(b) Kwashiorkor or pellagra.

178 (a) Coloboma of the iris.
(b) Patau's syndrome, Goldenhar's syndrome and Wolf's syndrome.

179 (a) Ritter's disease.
(b) Staphylococcal exotoxin.
(c) Parenteral cloxacillin and fusidic acid.

180 (a) The rash is a plexiform neurofibroma.
(b) Optic nerve glioma and buphthalmos.

181 (a) A yolk-sac tumour, otherwise known as an endodermal sinus tumour.
(b) Either pulmonary metastases or primary mediastinal involvement.

182 (a) Syndactyly of the third and fourth fingers.
(b) Apert's, Carpenter's or orofaciodigital syndromes.

183 (a) Scaphocephaly.
(b) Premature fusion of the sagittal suture.
(c) Surgical intervention may be indicated if early diagnosis is made.

184 (a) Ichthyosis.
(b) Refsum's syndrome.
(c) Avoidance of all green plant foods and other phytanic acid containing foods.

185 (a) The lesions are burns from application of a transcutaneous p0$_2$ monitor.
(b) Includes congenital chicken pox.

186 (a) Angioneurotic oedema.
(b) Adrenalin and/or systemic antihistamines.

187 (a) Shingles.
(b) Herpes zoster infection.
(c) Spontaneous resolution occurs after 7 to 14 days.

188 (a) Bilateral hilar enlargement, and generalised mottling of both pulmonary fields.
(b) Miliary tuberculosis.
(c) Mantoux test and gastric washings for acid fast bacilli.

189 (a) Pubic hair.
(b) Twenty-four-hour urinary steroid excretion, abdominal ultrasound, abdominal CAT scan and laparoscopy.

190 (a) Inflammation of the lips (cheilitis).
(b) This is seen in febrile illness, contact dermatitis or excess salivation.

191 (a) Embarrassment because of micropenis.
(b) The commonest explanation for this apparent finding is obesity. True micropenis is found in gonadotrophin deficiency and the Prader–Willi syndrome.

192 (a) A myelogram.
(b) Splitting of the lumbar spinal cord by a septum.
(c) A diastomatomyelia.

193 (a) Hydrocephalus.
(b) If it is progressive, treatment is surgical by means of a ventriculoatrial or ventriculoperitoneal shunt. Otherwise treatment is medical.
(c) 'Sunsetting' of the eyes, dilated scalp veins, a full fontanelle, separation of the sutures, optic atrophy, stridor.

194 (a) Supraventricular tachycardia.
(b) Wolff–Parkinson–White syndrome.

195 (a) Scalp skin defects.
(b) Patau's syndrome.
(c) The diagnosis may be confirmed by chromosomal analysis.

196 (a) A modified barium swallow.
(b) A flow of contrast medium into the trachea.
(c) H-type tracheo-oesophageal fistula.

197 (a) Pseudohypertrophy of the thigh and calf muscles and a lumbar lordosis.
(b) Duchenne's muscular dystrophy.
(c) X-linked recessive.

198 (a) Atypical mycobacterium infection.
(b) Excision possibly with antituberculous chemotherapy cover.

199 (a) Round face, hypertelorism, downward slanting eyes, and anteverted nares.
(b) Aarskog syndrome.

200 Hydrocephalus and agenesis of the cerebellar vermis and part of the right cerebellar hemisphere.